HEPATOLOGY RESEARCH AND CLINICAL DEVELOPMENTS

ALCOHOL AND THE LIVER

Hepatology Research and Clinical Developments

Additional books in this series can be found on Nova's website under the Series tab.

Additional e-books in this series can be found on Nova's website under the e-book tab.

HEPATOLOGY RESEARCH AND CLINICAL DEVELOPMENTS

ALCOHOL AND THE LIVER

GERONDLAKE-BAKAAR
EDITOR

NOVA BIOMEDICAL
New York

Library of Congress Cataloging-in-Publication Data

ISBN: 978-1-63484-400-0

Library of Congress Control Number: 2015959372

Published by Nova Science Publishers, Inc. † New York

CONTENTS

Preface		**vii**
Chapter 1	Alcohol Metabolism and Alcoholic Liver Disease *Gerond Lake-Bakaar*	**1**
Chapter 2	Inflammation in Alcoholic Liver Disease *Laura Hand and Mark A. Exley*	**17**
Chapter 3	Purinergic Signaling and the Inflammasome in Acute Alcoholic Liver Disease *Paola de Adrade Mello, Trishan Vaikunthanathan and Simon C. Robson*	**31**
Chapter 4	Assessment of Malnutrition in Alcoholic Liver Disease *Audrey Paradis*	**51**
Chapter 5	Vitamins and Supplements in Alcoholic Liver Disease *Katelyn R. Richards*	**63**
Chapter 6	Liver Transplantation for Alcoholic Liver Disease *Saikiran Kilaru and Michael P. Curry*	**79**
Chapter 7	Alcoholic and Nonalcoholic Fatty Liver Disease *Gary Trey*	**101**
Chapter 8	Pathologic Features and Mechanisms in Alcoholic Liver Disease *Imad A. Nasser*	**109**

Chapter 9 Alcohol and the Liver: Role of Mitochondria **119**
Alfredo Saavedra-Molina, Héctor Riveros-Rosas, Adriana Julián-Sánchez, Rocío Montoya-Pérez and Ruth Noriega-Cisneros

Editor's Contact Information **159**

Index **161**

PREFACE

The topic of alcohol and the liver is long overdue for re-evaluation. The authors of this book have clearly taken up this challenge.

Human interest in alcohol dates back to the Neolithic period (circa 10,000 BC). Only a small amount of alcohol is found naturally in food. Therefore, humans have yet to adapt to the high quantities of alcohol consumed daily by alcohol abusers.

Alcohol is a simple carbohydrate and is metabolized as a fuel. However, unlike more naturally occurring carbohydrates such as glucose, the pathways for its metabolism are not subject to the same checks and balances. Ethanol oxidation reduces NAD+, which starves reactions that depend on this substrate. This accounts for the accumulation of fat in alcoholic steatosis. Alcohol metabolism generates significant amounts of reactive oxygen species (ROS), which damages mtDNA and subsequently mitochondrial integrity. The authors provide several lines of evidence that link the clinical picture of alcoholic liver disease with mitochondrial damage. Other important topics highlighted in this book include histo-pathological aspects of the disease. Clinical assessment of nutrition and vitamin supplementation is addressed as well. The book concludes with the highly topical and controversial aspect of liver transplantation in patients with alcoholic liver disease.

Chapter 1 - Despite years of intensive study of alcoholic liver disease, the relationship between chronic ethanol consumption and the development and progression of alcoholic liver disease, remains unclear. Ethanol is a simple carbohydrate. However, its metabolism differs significantly from that of glucose.

This article reviews the impact of alcohol on glucose and fatty acid metabolism, much of which takes place in mitochondria. The metabolism of glucose and fatty acids is subject to multiple checks and balances that are governed by the accumulation and build up of metabolites. Many fewer feed-back loops have evolved for alcohol metabolism. As a consequence, chronic excessive ethanol consumption imposes significant stress on mitochondria. The authors suggest that this is what ultimately results in alcoholic liver disease. The article summarizes evidence supporting a direct effect of chronic alcohol abuse on the integrity of mitochondria.

The long latency between alcohol abuse and the onset of liver damage is explained by the high redundancy of functioning hepatocytes in the liver of hepatic reserve; the regenerative capacity of the hepatocytes; the redundancy of mitochondria in liver cells; and finally the redundancy of mitochondrial DNA, mtDNA, in individual mitochondria.

Evidence for structural mitochondrial damage is presented. Aspartate transaminase AST is largely present in mitochondria. By contrast, alanine transaminase ALT is largely cytosolic in origin. Thus, structural damage to mitochondria results in increased AST to ALT leakage into serum in alcoholic hepatitis.

Reactive oxygen species, ROS, generated by excess ethanol metabolism in mitochondria can damage the sensitive mtDNA. Consequent structural changes to mitochondrial membrane could lead to escape of cyt c. This triggers activation of caspases and invokes apoptosis. Cells that die as a result of apoptosis shrivel and contract allowing only modest leakage of enzymes into serum. This could explain the low levels of transaminases that are characteristic of alcoholic hepatitis.

These several observations argue for the involvement of mitochondria in the pathophysiology of alcohol-induced hepatotoxicity. They also raise questions about the use of immunosuppressive therapies in the treatment of alcoholic liver disease. The use of steroids and of tumor necrosis factor TNF inhibitors like pentoxifylline should be avoided as first line theapy in alcoholic hepatitis.

Chapter 2 - The liver processes and detoxifies toxins. It is also a barrier to pathogens absorbed from the gut via the portal circulatory system. Consequently, along with being the major metabolic organ, the liver contains a substantial population of immunologically active cells, including T and B lymphocytes, liver resident macrophages (Kupffer cells), natural killer (NK) cells, NKT cells, and dendritic cells, all of which are exposed to ingested toxins and pathogens.

Acute inflammation protects the host against tissue infection and injury. It is characterized by immune cell infiltration into target tissues to orchestrate the killing and removal of infected/damaged cells, and subsequently to promote tissue repair and regeneration. Chronic inflammation occurs when an acute response fails to resolve due to the continued presence of an inducer of inflammation and/or lack of normal immunoregulation. The excessive and persistent presence of cytotoxic immune cells and their mediators play important roles in the pathogenesis of human diseases, including alcoholic liver disease (ALD).

Several proinflammatory mediators that contribute to the development of ALD, against a background of failed immunoregulation have been proposed. The authors discuss their relative contributions to alcohol-mediated liver toxicity and inflammation.

Chapter 3 - Alcoholic liver disease (ALD) comprises a range of disorders including alcoholic fatty liver (steatosis), alcoholic steatohepatitis with or without fibrosis, cirrhosis and hepatocellular cancer. Acute alcoholic hepatitis is the most severe form of the disease with high mortality and limited treatment options. Liver inflammation is the main characteristic of acute hepatitis and plays a central role in ALD progression. Understanding ALD pathogenesis in the context of inflammation and hepatocellular dysfunction may provide new insights for the disease treatment as well as facilitate discovery of novel targets to control disease progression.

In this chapter, the authors highlight aspects of purinergic signaling and inflammasome activation as important components of hepatic pathophysiology in ALD. Inflammasomes are intracellular multiprotein complexes that mediate cellular response to exogenous and endogenous danger signals resulting in immune cell activation and recruitment. When activated by extracellular nucleotides e.g., ATP *via* type 2 purinergic receptors, by derivative nucleosides such as adenosine or penultimate metabolites uric acid, the inflammasome promotes capase-1 activation resulting in IL-1β and IL-18 maturation and release. Patients with ALD exhibit high levels of IL-1β, noted also in models of alcoholic hepatitis. Consequently there are links to inflammasome activation in ALD onset and progression. The authors review the studies that link inflammasome activation to manifestations of disease, such as steatosis, liver inflammation and fibrosis, in ALD. Precise mechanisms involved in ALD still need to be elucidated and therapeutic options explored.

Chapter 4 - Defining malnutrition in individuals with liver disease is a challenge. Many tools that are typically used to assess nutrition status are not reliable indicators and should be used with caution. This chapter explores the current methods of assessing nutrition status and offers insight into the appropriate assessment of malnutrition in patients with alcoholic liver disease.

Chapter 5 - Significant malnutrition in alcoholics is caused by reduced dietary intake as well as alternations in absorption of essential vitamins and nutrients. Malabsorption may be due to alcohol's direct effect on the small intestine inhibiting the absorption of amino acids, lipids and vitamins. A decrease in biliary output can also play a role in the malabsorption of fat soluble vitamins. However, if dietary intake is reconciled, the alternations in absorption normalize.

Chapter 6 - Though initially controversial, liver transplantation (LT) currently plays a vital role in definitive treatment for alcoholic cirrhosis, and is now one of the most common indications. Data are emerging that LT for severe alcoholic hepatitis that is unresponsive to medical management may also play a role, though it is more controversial. The main concern in alcoholic patients is risk of relapse, and post-transplant interventions have been shown to reduce recidivism. Special considerations for patients transplanted for alcoholic liver disease center around post-transplant interventions to improve mortality, such as tobacco cessation and surveillance for malignancy.

Chapter 7 - Excess calorie consumption and excessive ingestion of alcohol are prevalent. Both can lead to fat accumulation in the liver and can progress to liver fibrosis, cirrhosis and hepatocellular carcinoma. When the two diseases coexist in the same individual the chances of progression are increased.

Many patients will have risk factors for both conditions and therefore may have both diseases, but these diseases are difficult to distinguish because of the similar histology. This chapter discusses each entity and addresses possible interactions in the clinical presentation.

Chapter 8 - Chronic alcohol abuse is a cause of significant mobidity and mortality in the US and other countries. The liver is one of the major organs affected. This chapter addresses the pathological changes in alcoholic liver disease.

Alcohol induced liver injury progresses from simple steatosis to steatohepatitis with perisinusoidal fibrosis and finally to cirrhosis. About 20%-30% of patients with steatosis develop alcoholic hepatitis and 16% of patients with steatohepatitis progress to cirrhosis.

The authors discuss specific forms of presentation of alcoholic liver disease. As an example, foamy degeneration is a rare lesion characterized by hepatocytes filled with small fat droplets with increase in size of the cells.

Potential mechanisms of alcohol induced liver injury are also discussed.

In: Alcohol and the Liver
Editor: Gerond Lake-Bakaar ISBN: 978-1-63484-400-0

Chapter 1

ALCOHOL METABOLISM AND ALCOHOLIC LIVER DISEASE

Gerond Lake-Bakaar**, *MD, PhD
Director, Liver Tumor Center, Beth Israel Deaconess Medical Center
Associate Professor of Medicine, Harvard Medical School,
Boston, MA, US

ABSTRACT

Despite years of intensive study of alcoholic liver disease, the relationship between chronic ethanol consumption and the development and progression of alcoholic liver disease, remains unclear. Ethanol is a simple carbohydrate. However, its metabolism differs significantly from that of glucose.

This article reviews the impact of alcohol on glucose and fatty acid metabolism, much of which takes place in mitochondria. The metabolism of glucose and fatty acids is subject to multiple checks and balances that are governed by the accumulation and build up of metabolites. Many fewer feed-back loops have evolved for alcohol metabolism. As a consequence, chronic excessive ethanol consumption imposes significant stress on mitochondria. We suggest that this is what ultimately results in

* Gerond Lake-Bakaar, MD, PhD: Director, Liver Tumor Center, Beth Israel Deaconess Medical Center. Associate Professor of Medicine, Harvard Medical School, 110 Francis Street, LMOB 7A-055, Boston, MA 01770.

alcoholic liver disease. The article summarizes evidence supporting a direct effect of chronic alcohol abuse on the integrity of mitochondria.

The long latency between alcohol abuse and the onset of liver damage is explained by the high redundancy of functioning hepatocytes in the liver of hepatic reserve; the regenerative capacity of the hepatocytes; the redundancy of mitochondria in liver cells; and finally the redundancy of mitochondrial DNA, mtDNA, in individual mitochondria.

Evidence for structural mitochondrial damage is presented. Aspartate transaminase AST is largely present in mitochondria. By contrast, alanine transaminase ALT is largely cytosolic in origin. Thus, structural damage to mitochondria results in increased AST to ALT leakage into serum in alcoholic hepatitis.

Reactive oxygen species, ROS, generated by excess ethanol metabolism in mitochondria can damage the sensitive mtDNA. Consequent structural changes to mitochondrial membrane could lead to escape of cyt c. This triggers activation of caspases and invokes apoptosis. Cells that die as a result of apoptosis shrivel and contract allowing only modest leakage of enzymes into serum. This could explain the low levels of transaminases that are characteristic of alcoholic hepatitis.

These several observations argue for the involvement of mitochondria in the pathophysiology of alcohol-induced hepatotoxicity. They also raise questions about the use of immunosuppressive therapies in the treatment of alcoholic liver disease. The use of steroids and of tumor necrosis factor TNF inhibitors like pentoxifylline should be avoided as first line therapy in alcoholic hepatitis.

INTRODUCTION

Despite years of intensive study of alcoholic liver disease, the relationship between chronic ethanol consumption and the development and progression of alcoholic liver disease, remains controversial.

Chronic consumption of excessive amounts of alcohol causes injury mainly to organs that contain a high copy number of cellular mitochondria. These include the liver, pancreas, nerves, muscle and bone marrow. Alcohol is metabolized mainly in the liver. Within each hepatic lobule, toxicity is confined largely to the hepatocytes surrounding the central veins. The enzymes associated with alcohol metabolism are mostly concentrated in this area [1, 2]. Thus, alcoholic hepatotoxicity may be associated with its metabolism in the liver and perhaps, more specifically to its oxidation in mitochondria [3, 4].

Mitochondria are considered to be the powerhouse of cells. They oxidize nutrients and in the process, generate energy. Compared to other organs, mitochondria have a unique role in the liver. They participate in the metabolism of all food components, carbohydrates, lipids and proteins [5].

Alcohol is a simple carbohydrate, C_2H_5OH. It is less than half the size of the glucose molecule, $C_6H_{12}O_6$. Alcohol is converted in the cytosol to acetaldehyde by the enzyme alcohol dehydrogenase ALD. Acetaldehyde is then transported to mitochondria and converted to acetate by aldehyde dehydrogenase ALDH. Both oxidizing reactions require NAD^+, which is converted to NADH.

By contrast, glucose is converted within the cytosol to pyruvate, $C_3H_4O_3$ via the 10-step glycolytic pathway. This process, like alcohol oxidation requires NAD^+, which is similarly converted to NADH. Pyruvate, like acetaldehyde is transported from the cytosol into the mitochondria, where it is oxidized into acetyl-Co-A. This process also requires NAD^+, with subsequent reduction to NADH. Thus, alcohol and glucose metabolism compete for NAD^+. Acetyl-Co-A can be further oxidized via the TCA cycle in the mitochondria to yield energy in the form of ATP, carbon dioxide and water. If energy is not immediately required, or when NADH levels are increased, acetyl-Co-A can be reduced to fatty acids and fats for storage [6].

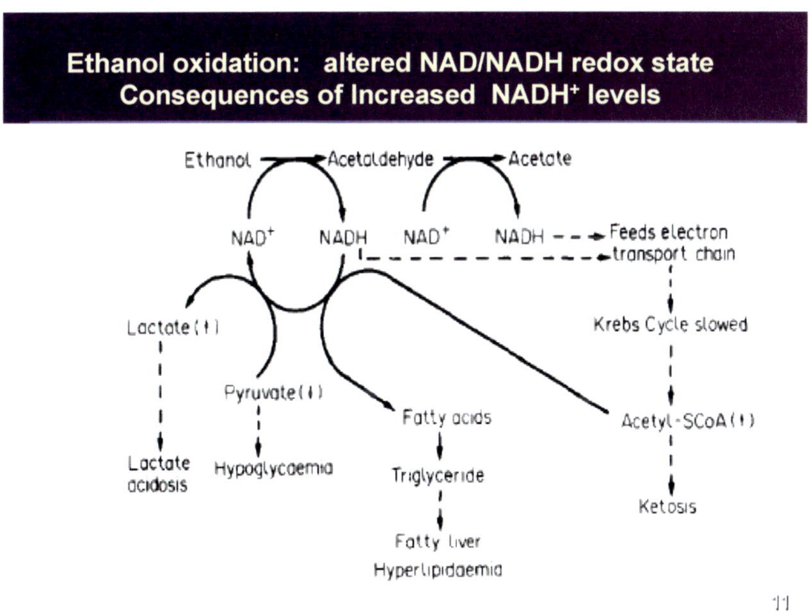

The oxidation of alcohol is associated with a reduction in NAD^+ and an increase in NADH. The reduced NAD^+ in the cell can impact glucose metabolism. Similarly, increased NADH favors fatty acid synthesis leading to fat accumulation [7].

Mitochondrial electron transport is a major source of reactive oxygen species ROS. Alcohol imposes conditions that promote ROS. Increased ROS generation as a result of chronic alcohol metabolism can result in mitochondrial damage and begin to explain alcoholic liver disease pathophysiology [8].

Alcohol Metabolism

Approximately 20 percent of ingested alcohol is passively absorbed across the gastric mucosa. The remainder is absorbed in the duodenum and small intestine. Gastric alcohol dehydrogenase is capable of metabolizing a small fraction of alcohol in the stomach wall. This enzyme is present at lower concentrations in women and could account for observed gender differences in alcohol absorption and first pass metabolism [9, 10]. Nearly all of the absorbed alcohol is eliminated by metabolism in the liver; just over 1 percent is excreted unchanged in breath, sweat and urine.

Alcohol Metabolism in the Liver

The enzymes associated with alcohol metabolism are concentrated in the centrilobular area or zone 3 [11].

In non-alcoholics, ethanol (C_2H_5OH) is oxidized to acetaldehyde (CH_3CHO) in a reversible reaction catalyzed by alcohol dehydrogenase ADH, in the cytosol of the liver cell. ADH has high affinity ($Km = 0.05\text{-}0.1$ g/L), but low capacity for ethanol and is readily saturated.

In chronic alcohol consumption, a second pathway, microsomal ethanol-oxidizing system (MEOS) is induced [12, 13]. This function resides in the smooth endoplasmic reticulum, SER, of the hepatocytes and works through the cytochrome P450 system (CYP2E1). Like ADH, it converts alcohol to acetaldehyde. The reaction requires oxygen. Unlike ADH, which reduces NAD to NADH, the reaction involves oxidation of reduced NADPH, which is converted to NADP and water. Cytochrome P450 is a highly inducible enzyme system that is widely used in drug catabolism. Chronic alcohol consumption leads to marked proliferation of SER in hepatocytes.

A third pathway involves catalase, which is located in cell bodies called peroxisomes [14]. It can oxidize a small amount of alcohol, approximately two percent, in the presence of hydrogen peroxide, H_2O_2, to acetaldehyde. This reaction does not need NAD as a cofactor.

Acetaldehyde produced in the cytosol is subsequently transported to, and oxidized in the mitochondria to acetate (CH_3COOH), in a non-reversible reaction by aldehyde dehydrogenase (ALDH). Acetaldehyde is highly toxic and needs to be eliminated rapidly [15]. Therefore, in contrast to ADH, ALDH has a low Km and efficiently eliminates acetaldehyde.

Alcohol Dehydrogenase and Acetaldehyde Dehydrogenase

Alcohol dehydrogenase ADH and acetaldehyde dehydrogenase ALDH are expressed at their highest concentrations in the liver, but lower levels are present in other tissue. They metabolize most of the alcohol ingested. It is likely that these enzymes evolved to detoxify small quantities of alcohol present in food.

Polymorphic variants of the genes for these enzymes encode proteins with different kinetic properties that may possess potential clinical relevance. ADH variants with high activity and ALDH variants with low activity may both result in high acetaldehyde accumulation [16].

ADH variants are all dimeric, zinc containing metalloproteinases, each subunit with a molecular weight of 40 kDa. A new nomenclature has introduced six classes of enzymes. The ADH beta2 encoded by the ADH2*2gene has high activity, increases acetaldehyde production and has been associated with a reduced risk of alcoholism.

ALDH are tetrameric enzymes, composed of 54 kDA subunits. They have been tentatively classified as class 1 (low Km, cytosolic), class 2 (low Km, mitochondrial) and class 3 (high Km, expressed in tumors, cornea and stomach) There are significant differences in the distribution across racial groups. Almost 50 percent of Japanese and Chinese are deficient in ALDH2 and most flush with alcohol ingestion. The mutation for the deficiency is a G to A substitution at position 487 in ALDH2, resulting in replacement of glutamate with lysine. The wild allele is the ALDH2*1 and the mutant allele,

ALDH2*2. The mutant allele has essentially no ALDH2 activity. This deficiency is almost absent in the Negro and Caucasian populations.

ADH and ALDH variants have been extensively studied for possible association with alcoholic liver disease and multiple other disease states including cancer and fetal alcohol syndrome. The strongest correlation has been between the ALDH2*2 allele and cancers of the oropharynx and esophagus. No association has been found with alcoholic liver disease [16].

Alcohol and Biochemical Homeostasis

Alcohol is a simple carbohydrate molecule and its metabolism involves relatively simple oxidative pathways. Nevertheless, alcohol consumption can significantly affect other biochemical pathways, especially when consumed chronically and in excess. Products generated during alcohol metabolism can profoundly influence biochemical homeostasis.

Oxidation of alcohol to acetaldehyde by ADH, and of acetaldehyde to acetate by ALDH, both require reduction of NAD^+ to NADH. This increases the ratio of NADH to NAD^+ in the cell. As a consequence, reactions that are driven by NADH are promoted. Such reactions include anaerobic conversion of pyruvate derived from glycolysis to lactate. Large quantities of lactic acid can accumulate in the cell and lead to metabolic acidosis. At the same time, especially in malnourished alcoholics with depleted glycogen levels, hypoglycemia can result from the reduced levels of pyruvate [17, 18].

Fats are generally stored as triglycerides. Breakdown of triglycerides by lipase yields three fatty acids and glycerol. During the oxidation of fatty acids, NAD^+ is reduced to NADH. The high NADH and low amounts of NAD^+ inhibits fatty acid oxidation and favors synthesis and formation of triglycerides, resulting in the accumulation of fat in the liver [7].

Alcohol and Net Energy Production

Glucose is the major source of fuel for the body. In the process of glycolysis leading to the formation of pyruvate, there is net production of two ATP and two NADH molecules.

Oxidation of pyruvate takes place via the Kreb's or citric acid (Tri-carboxylic acid) cycle in the mitochondria. The overall objective is conversion of pyruvate formed from glycolysis to acetyl-CoA in mitochondria. There are several intermediary steps. The net result is that the six-carbon backbone of pyruvate is reduced to two in acetyl-CoA and four molecules of carbon dioxide. A total of two ATP molecules as well as six NADH and two $FADH_2$ molecules that can later be converted to ATP via the electron transport chain are released. In the final analysis, one glucose molecule produces a total of 10 NADH (30 ATP), two FADH2 (four ATP) and four ATP molecules. All six carbon atoms are oxidized and released from the cell as waste and a total of 38 ATP molecules are produced.

As we have demonstrated above, the metabolism of alcohol is associated with increased $NADH/NAD^+$ ratio. Thus, the several intermediary steps in the Kreb's cycle that require NAD^+ will be inhibited in the presence of alcohol metabolism. The major site of inhibition is at the alpha-ketoglutarate oxidation step of the Kreb's cycle, with minor inhibition between succinate and citrate. In the intact liver cell, ethanol inhibits the TCA cycle by approximately 20–30 percent [7].

Mitochondria and Alcoholic Liver Disease

Most of the energy-producing molecules generated as a result of ethanol or glucose metabolism arise in mitochondria. An understanding of how alcohol metabolism influences mitochondrial function is therefore vital to our understanding of the potential mechanisms by which alcohol induces liver damage.

As we show later, mitochondrial damage induced by excessive alcohol consumption could account for many of the changes associated with alcoholic liver disease [8].

Mitochondria Structure

Mitochondria are organelles with a double membrane structure found in most eukaryotic cells. Between the inner and outer membranes is the intermediate space. The inner membrane encloses the mitochondrial matrix. The number of mitochondria in each cell varies according to the energy requirements of that cell. Liver, muscle, nerves and pancreas are particularly rich in mitochondria [19]. Hepatocytes contain approximately 800 mitochondria per cell and these occupy about 18 percent of the cell [8].

The inner membrane has a highly complex structure. It comprises all the constituents of the electron transport system, the ATP synthase complex and a number of transport proteins. The mitochondrial matrix contains a mixture of enzymes involved in pyruvate and fatty acid oxidation in the Kreb's cycle. The matrix also contains mitochondrial DNA (mtDNA) genomes sequestered in distinct compartments. Human mtDNA consists of 13 structural genes, which encode for subunits of the respiratory complexes I, III, IV and V of the respiratory chain involved in ATP generation [20, 21].

There is a high redundancy of mtDNA copies in each mitochondrion and of mitochondria in each cell. Each mitochondrion contains between five to ten copies of mtDNA. It is estimated that the number of mtDNA copies per cell has to fall below 20 percent to 40 percent of the basal levels to induce mitochondrial dysfunction in the cell [22].

Unlike nuclear DNA, the mtDNA repair system is incomplete. It is very sensitive to reactive oxygen species (ROS) induced oxidative damage, since it docs not contain histones and because it is close to the inner mitochondrial membrane that is the source of most of the ROS in the cell.

Mitochondria in the liver participate in the metabolism of all food groups: carbohydrates (glucose), lipids and proteins. Oxidation of acetyl-CoA via Kreb's cycle generates reduced NADH and reduced FADH2 (flavine-adenine-dinucleotide), which transfer the hydrogen/electron to an oxygen molecule via several redox components in complex I through IV, in the mitochondrial respiratory chain. The flow of electrons in the respiratory chain, located in the inner mitochondrial membrane, is coupled with the pumping of protons from the mitochondrial matrix into the inter-membrane space, creating a pH gradient and an electrical potential difference across the inner membrane that together constitute the proton motive force. This proton motive force is the driving force for ATP synthesis through the proton pumping ATP synthase. The process of oxidation via the Kreb's cycle, linked to the production of ATP is known as oxidative phosphorylation.

The rate of oxidation of NADH via the electron transport chain is limited by the cellular need for ATP. Regulatory mechanisms link the demand for ATP to the oxidation of substrates. When ATP levels are low, protons re-enter the matrix through ATP synthase and the energy released, generates ATP synthesis.

The cell can also relax the strict coupling of substrate oxidation to ATP formation using uncoupling proteins, which allow leakage of protons across the mitochondrial membrane, allowing electron transport without ATP formation. Excessive electron flow to the respiratory chain can result in accumulation and leakage of electrons at complex I and II, where insulation from oxygen is not perfect. This can result in increased ROS production through reduction of oxygen to superoxide O2- by complex I and III [23-25].

Excessive production of ROS can damage components of the mitochondria including the membrane and mtDNA. This is particularly relevant in conditions of increased FFA oxidation, such as NASH (non alcoholic steatohepatitis) or when NADH levels are increased as during alcohol metabolism [26-29].

Chronic Alcohol Consumption, Mitochondrial Structure and mtDNA

Chronic alcohol consumption has been associated with changes in mitochondrial structure and function. In the liver cells, mitochondria are enlarged and distorted. Megamitochondria can be detected as early as the fatty liver stage. Changes in both the protein and lipid content of the mitochondrial membranes have also been described [30].

It is not clear to what extent damage to the integrity of the mtDNA by ethanol affects cell function. The effect on encoded proteins could impair mitochondrial structure and function. This in turn might influence global cell function and cause tissue injury. Chronic exposure to high acetaldehyde levels can also cause long-term tissue damage. Acetaldehyde is very reactive chemically, and has a number of toxic effects [31].

Typically, alcoholic liver disease becomes clinically apparent only after several years of excessive alcohol abuse. The prolonged latency between the initiation of alcohol abuse and the onset of clinical liver disease could be explained by damage to mtDNA and subsequent effects on direct mitochondrial structure and function. Approximately 60%-80% of the mitochondria and mtDNA are redundant or surplus to requirements. Therefore, the liver cell can tolerate injury to a significant number of mtDNA and mitochondria before it succumbs.

There are a number of alternative hypotheses for alcoholic liver disease. One of the more popular is based on studies in animal models. It suggests that alcohol induces gut permeability, which in turn increases absorption of gut-derived endotoxins. The theory relates alcoholic liver disease to the endotoxins

[32-34]. Another is that alcohol triggers an immune reaction that persists in the absence of the offending toxin [32-34]. Unfortunately, neither explains the prolonged latency, up to 10 years, between initiation of alcohol abuse and the onset of alcoholic liver disease. They also fail to account for the perivenular distribution of alcoholic liver disease.

Thus far, we have suggested that alcohol hepatoxicity might be related to its metabolism by mitochondria in the liver. The associated generation of ROS induces damage to mtDNA and subsequently to mitochondria, both of which are present with high redundancy in the liver. The structural changes in mitochondria induced by alcohol [4, 36, 37] and the redundancy of these organelles, explains in part, the long latency between alcohol abuse and the onset of clinical alcoholic liver disease. We believe that the mode of death of hepatocytes in alcoholic liver disease, by a process known as apoptosis can also be linked to mitochondria.

Apoptosis

The outer mitochondrial cell and the intermembrane space are intimately involved in the process of apoptosis, or programmed cell death. A family of proteins related to the Bcl-2 oncogene, regulate apoptosis. Bcl-2 and Bcl-X_L protect the cell from apoptosis. By contrast, Bax, Bad and Bid enhance the process of programmed cell death. The balance between pro- and anti-apoptotic proteins determines the fate of the cell [35].

The Bcl-2 proteins interact with the mitochondrial membranes, resulting in release of proteins sequestered in the mitochondrial space. These proteins include cytochrome c, which acts as a co-factor for activation of the protease caspase 9. The activated protein migrates to the nucleus and activates endonucleases.

In general, apoptosis serves to dispose of damaged cells and cellular debris. It is not harmful to the organism. Approximately 50-70 billion cells in the body die from apoptosis each day. In apoptosis, the cell shrinks, the cytoplasm appears dense and the organelles become tightly packed. Pyknosis is characteristic and is the result of chromatin condensation. It involves single cells or small clusters of cells [35].

The alternative process to apoptosis is necrosis. This involves cell swelling with disruption and rupture of lysosomes with eventual rupture of the cell membrane. The cytoplasmic content is released into surrounding tissue and extracellular fluid with eventual recruitment of inflammatory cells.

Apoptotic cells by contrast do not release their content into interstitial tissue and are quickly phagocytized by macrophages with essentially no inflammatory reaction [38].

Clinical Presentation of Alcoholic Liver Disease

In alcoholic liver disease the activity of aspartate aminotransferase, AST, in serum is characteristically higher and often at twice that of alanine aminotransferase ALT. Aspartate amino-transaminase originates predominantly from mitochondria [39]. In contrast, alanine amino-transaminase is found mainly in the cytosol [40]. The higher levels of the former in serum of patient with alcoholic hepatitis, more likely indicates structural damage to mitochondria.

The increase in AST elevation is modest and characteristically, rarely exceeds 300 iu/ml. This is indicative of cell death by apoptosis, in which cells shrink and the contents become condensed. Alcoholic hepatitis contrasts sharply from other types of liver disease such as viral hepatitis, where ALT elevation predominates and where the levels are much higher, suggesting cell swelling and rupture with release of contents into the surrounding tissue [38].

There is a prolonged latency between alcohol consumption and onset of clinical evidence of disease. Alcoholic liver disease generally follows alcohol abuse over several years. On average, it requires 10 years of consuming at least 30g a day of ethanol in females and 40 g in males. This is the equivalent of consuming approximately twice the average body weight of alcohol. The prolonged latency implies damage to organelle(s) present with high redundancy in the liver cell [22]. It probably also reflects the high regenerative potential of hepatocytes. Dying liver cells are readily replaced by regenerating hepatocytes.

Histologically, liver cell damage in alcoholic liver disease is usual concentrated in the perivenular area, or zone 3. The enzymes responsible for alcohol metabolism, alcohol dehydrogenase and acetaldehyde dehydrogenase are located in highest concentration in this area [41]. Interestingly, acetaldehyde dehydrogenase is also present mainly in mitochondria.

Circulating levels of Cytokeratin 18 (CK18) and its caspase-generated fragments have been correlated with disease severity in heavy alcoholics. Serum levels of markers of hepatocyte death (CK18) and apoptosis (CK18 fragment) are increased in patients with severe fibrosis compared to patients with mild fibrosis. These markers also strongly correlate with Mallory-Denk bodies [42]. Increased TdT labeling of hepatocytes [43] and expression of apoptosis-related Lewis(Le)(y) antigen by immunohistochemistry [44], both of which indicate apoptotic bodies, have been demonstrated in patients with alcoholic liver disease.

Another characteristic, clinical feature of alcoholic hepatitis is that serum direct bilirubin levels and other evidence of progressing hepatocyte death continue to worsen for some time, even after all contact with alcohol has been removed. This frequently noted clinical observation is unexplained. A probable explanation is continued deterioration of damaged mitochondria and subsequent death of hepatocytes. The cells die as mtDNA impairment progresses and the number of mitochondria in the cells fall. As the balance between regenerating and dying cells is reversed, the bilirubin levels start to fall. This downward change in bilirubin level usually indicates the advent of clinical recovery.

Conclusion

Several features associated with the natural history of alcoholic hepatitis suggest that hepatotoxicity might be due to mitochondria damage from alcohol metabolism and associated generation of ROS.

Chronic alcohol abuse and attendant alcohol metabolism results in the generation of excessive reactive oxygen species ROS. Damage to mtDNA and mitochondria structure is consistent with the clinical development of hepatic steatosis, alcoholic hepatitis and progressive alcoholic liver disease. Against this background, the use of pentoxifylline and of steroids, especially given the increased risk of infection, warrants caution. Indeed, recently published data on the survival of patients treated with pentoxifylline or steroids argues against their routine use in alcoholic hepatitis [45].

References

[1] Ito, D., Ishii, H., Kato, S., Takagi, T., Takekawa, S., Aiso, S. et al. Significance of alcohol dehydrogenase (ADH) as a marker of hepatic centrilobular injury: a biochemical and immunohistochemical study. *Alcohol Alcohol. Suppl.* 1987;1:523-7.

[2] Kato, S., Ishii, H., Kano, S., Hagihara, S., Todoroki, T., Nagata, S. et al. Alcohol dehydrogenase: a new sensitive marker of hepatic centrilobular damage. *Alcohol*. 1985;2(1):35-8.

[3] Garcia-Ruiz, C., Morales, A., Ballesta, A., Rodes, J., Kaplowitz, N., Fernandez-Checa, J. C. Effect of chronic ethanol feeding on glutathione and functional integrity of mitochondria in periportal and perivenous rat hepatocytes. *J. Clin. Invest*. 1994;94(1):193-201.

[4] French, S. W., Ruebner, B. H., Mezey, E., Tamura, T., Halsted, C. H. Effect of chronic ethanol feeding on hepatic mitochondria in the monkey. *Hepatology*. 1983;3(1):34-40.

[5] Rui, L. Energy metabolism in the liver. *Compr. Physiol*. 2014;4(1):177-97.

[6] Dashty, M. A quick look at biochemistry: carbohydrate metabolism. *Clin. Biochem*. 2013;46(15):1339-52.

[7] Ontko, J. A. Effects of ethanol on the metabolism of free fatty acids in isolated liver cells. *J. Lipid Res*. 1973;14(1):78-86.

[8] Hoek, J. B., Cahill, A., Pastorino, J. G. Alcohol and mitochondria: a dysfunctional relationship. *Gastroenterology*. 2002;122(7):2049-63.

[9] Baraona, E., Abittan, C. S., Dohmen, K., Moretti, M., Pozzato, G., Chayes, Z. W. et al. Gender differences in pharmacokinetics of alcohol. *Alcohol. Clin. Exp. Res*. 2001;25(4):502-7.

[10] Frezza, M., di Padova, C., Pozzato, G., Terpin, M., Baraona, E., Lieber, C. S. High blood alcohol levels in women. The role of decreased gastric alcohol dehydrogenase activity and first-pass metabolism. *N. Engl. J. Med*. 1990;322(2):95-9.

[11] Forkert, P. G., Massey, T. E., Jones, A. B., Park, S. S., Gelboin, H. V., Anderson, L. M. Distribution of cytochrome CYP2E1 in murine liver after ethanol and acetone administration. *Carcinogenesis*. 1991;12(12): 2259-68.

[12] Lieber, C. S. The discovery of the microsomal ethanol oxidizing system and its physiologic and pathologic role. *Drug Metab. Rev*. 2004;36(3-4): 511-29.

[13] Djordjevic, D., Nikolic, J., Stefanovic, V. Ethanol interactions with other cytochrome P450 substrates including drugs, xenobiotics, and carcinogens. *Pathol. Biol*. (Paris). 1998;46(10):760-70.

[14] Bradford, B. U., Enomoto, N., Ikejima, K., Rose, M. L., Bojes, H. K., Forman, D. T. et al. Peroxisomes are involved in the swift increase in alcohol metabolism. *J. Pharmacol. Exp. Ther*. 1999;288(1):254-9.

[15] Mello, T., Ceni, E., Surrenti, C., Galli, A. Alcohol induced hepatic fibrosis: role of acetaldehyde. *Mol. Aspects Med.* 2008;29(1-2):17-21.
[16] Crabb, D. W., Matsumoto, M., Chang, D., You, M. Overview of the role of alcohol dehydrogenase and aldehyde dehydrogenase and their variants in the genesis of alcohol-related pathology. *Proc. Nutr. Soc.* 2004;63(1): 49-63.
[17] Platia, E. V., Hsu, T. H. Hypoglycemic coma with ketoacidosis in nondiabetic alcoholics. *West. J. Med.* 1979;131(4):270-6.
[18] Halperin, M. L., Hammeke, M., Josse, R. G., Jungas, R. L. Metabolic acidosis in the alcoholic: a pathophysiologic approach. *Metabolism.* 1983;32(3):308-15.
[19] Perkins, G. A., Sun, M. G., Frey, T. G. Chapter 2 Correlated light and electron microscopy/electron tomography of mitochondria in situ. *Methods Enzymol.* 2009;456:29-52.
[20] Logan, D. C. The mitochondrial compartment. *J. Exp. Bot.* 2007;58(1): 1225-43.
[21] Kuroiwa, T., Nishida, K., Yoshida, Y., Fujiwara, T., Mori, T., Kuroiwa, H. et al. Structure, function and evolution of the mitochondrial division apparatus. *Biochim. Biophys. Acta.* 2006;1763(5-6):510-21.
[22] DiMauro, S., Schon, E. A. Mitochondrial DNA mutations in human disease. *Am. J. Med. Genet.* 2001;106(1):18-26.
[23] Lee, H. C., Wei, Y. H. Mitochondria and aging. *Adv. Exp. Med. Biol.* 2012;942:311-27.
[24] Fellman, V., Kotarsky, H. Mitochondrial hepatopathies in the newborn period. *Semin. Fetal Neonatal Med.* 2011;16(4):222-8.
[25] Wong, L. J. Molecular genetics of mitochondrial disorders. *Dev. Disabil. Res. Rev.* 2010;16(2):154-62.
[26] Pessayre, D., Mansouri, A., Haouzi, D., Fromenty, B. Hepatotoxicity due to mitochondrial dysfunction. *Cell Biol. Toxicol.* 1999;15(6):367-73.
[27] Cunningham, C. C., Bailey, S. M. Ethanol consumption and liver mitochondria function. *Biol. Signals Recept.* 2001;10(3-4):271-82.
[28] Adachi, M., Brenner, D. A. Clinical syndromes of alcoholic liver disease. *Dig. Dis.* 2005;23(3-4):255-63.
[29] Lemasters, J. J., Qian, T., He, L., Kim, J. S., Elmore, S. P., Cascio, W. E. et al. Role of mitochondrial inner membrane permeabilization in necrotic cell death, apoptosis, and autophagy. *Antioxid. Redox Signal.* 2002;4(5): 769-81.
[30] Gordon, E. R. Alcohol-induced mitochondrial changes in the liver. *Recent Dev. Alcohol.* 1984;2:143-58.

[31] Worrall, S., de Jersey, J., Nicholls, R., Wilce, P. Acetaldehyde/protein interactions: are they involved in the pathogenesis of alcoholic liver disease? *Dig. Dis.* 1993;11(4-5):265-77.

[32] Bode, C., Bode, J. C. Activation of the innate immune system and alcoholic liver disease: effects of ethanol per se or enhanced intestinal translocation of bacterial toxins induced by ethanol? *Alcohol. Clin. Exp. Res.* 2005;29(11 Suppl.):166S-71S.

[33] Chiu, W. C., Huang, Y. L., Chen, Y. L., Peng, H. C., Liao, W. H., Chuang, H. L. et al. Synbiotics reduce ethanol-induced hepatic steatosis and inflammation by improving intestinal permeability and microbiota in rats. *Food Funct.* 2015;6(5):1692-700.

[34] Nagata, K., Suzuki, H., Sakaguchi, S. Common pathogenic mechanism in development progression of liver injury caused by non-alcoholic or alcoholic steatohepatitis. *J. Toxicol. Sci.* 2007;32(5):453-68.

[35] Elmore, S. Apoptosis: a review of programmed cell death. *Toxicol. Pathol.* 2007;35(4):495-516.

[36] Chedid, A., Mendenhall, C. L., Tosch, T., Chen, T., Rabin, L., Garcia-Pont, P. et al. Significance of megamitochondria in alcoholic liver disease. *Gastroenterology.* 1986;90(6):1858-64.

[37] Uchida, T., Kao, H., Quispe-Sjogren, M., Peters, R. L. Alcoholic foamy degeneration--a pattern of acute alcoholic injury of the liver. *Gastroenterology.* 1983;84(4):683-92.

[38] Kurosaka, K., Kobayashi, Y. [Macrophage responses during phagocytosis of apoptotic cells and their regulatory mechanism]. *Seikagaku.* 2003;75(1):59-62.

[39] Okuno, F., Ishii, H., Kashiwazaki, K., Takagi, S., Shigeta, Y., Arai, M. et al. Increase in mitochondrial GOT (m-GOT) activity after chronic alcohol consumption: clinical and experimental observations. *Alcohol.* 1988;5(1):49-53.

[40] Yang, M., Antoine, D. J., Weemhoff, J. L., Jenkins, R. E., Farhood, A., Park, B. K. et al. Biomarkers distinguish apoptotic and necrotic cell death during hepatic ischemia/reperfusion injury in mice. *Liver Transpl.* 2014;20(11):1372-82.

[41] Maly, I. P., Toranelli, M., Sasse, D. Distribution of alcohol dehydrogenase isoenzymes in the human liver acinus. *Histochem. Cell Biol.* 1999;111(5):391-7.

[42] Lavallard, V. J., Bonnafous, S., Patouraux, S., Saint-Paul, M. C., Rousseau, D., Anty, R. et al. Serum markers of hepatocyte death and

apoptosis are non invasive biomarkers of severe fibrosis in patients with alcoholic liver disease. *PLoS One*. 2011;6(3):e17599.

[43] Zhao, M., Laissue, J. A., Zimmermann, A. TUNEL-positive hepatocytes in alcoholic liver disease. A retrospective biopsy study using DNA nick end-labelling. *Virchows Arch*. 1997;431(5):337-44.

[44] Kawahara, H., Matsuda, Y., Takase, S. Is apoptosis involved in alcoholic hepatitis? *Alcohol Alcohol*. Suppl. 1994;29(1):113-8.

[45] Thursz, M. R., Richardson, P., Allison, M., Austin, A., Bowers, M., Day, C. P. et al. Prednisolone or pentoxifylline for alcoholic hepatitis. *N. Engl. J. Med*. 2015;372(17):1619-28.

In: Alcohol and the Liver
Editor: Gerond Lake-Bakaar
ISBN: 978-1-63484-400-0

Chapter 2

INFLAMMATION IN ALCOHOLIC LIVER DISEASE

Laura Hand[1], PhD, and Mark A. Exley[1,2,*], PhD
[1]Manchester Collaborative Centre for Inflammation Research, University of Manchester, Manchester, UK
[2]Gastroenterology, Brigham and Women's Hospital, Harvard Medical School, Boston, MA, US

ABSTRACT

The liver processes and detoxifies toxins. It is also a barrier to pathogens absorbed from the gut via the portal circulatory system. Consequently, along with being the major metabolic organ, the liver contains a substantial population of immunologically active cells, including T and B lymphocytes, liver resident macrophages (Kupffer cells), natural killer (NK) cells, NKT cells, and dendritic cells, all of which are exposed to ingested toxins and pathogens.

Acute inflammation protects the host against tissue infection and injury. It is characterized by immune cell infiltration into target tissues to orchestrate the killing and removal of infected/damaged cells, and subsequently to promote tissue repair and regeneration. Chronic inflammation occurs when an acute response fails to resolve due to the

* Corresponding author: Professor Mark A. Exley, 75 Francis St., Thorn 1405, Boston, MA 02115. E-mail: mexley @partners.org, mark.exley@manchester.ac.uk.

continued presence of an inducer of inflammation and/or lack of normal immunoregulation. The excessive and persistent presence of cytotoxic immune cells and their mediators play important roles in the pathogenesis of human diseases, including alcoholic liver disease (ALD).

Several proinflammatory mediators that contribute to the development of ALD, against a background of failed immunoregulation have been proposed. We discuss their relative contributions to alcohol-mediated liver toxicity and inflammation.

ALCOHOL AND THE LIVER – INFLAMMATION IN ALCOHOLIC LIVER DISEASE

When extraneous molecules enter the body, they have to be processed by the liver, either by metabolism or detoxification. Therefore, the liver is a barrier against toxins and nutrients, as well as pathogens absorbed from the gut via the portal circulatory system.

Consequently, along with being the major metabolic organ, the liver contains a substantial population of immunologically active cells, including T and B lymphocytes, liver resident macrophages (Kupffer cells), natural killer (NK) cells, NKT cells, and dendritic cells, all of which are exposed to ingested toxins.

Acute inflammation is a critical mechanism for protecting the host against infection and tissue injury. Such inflammation, whether infectious or sterile in origin, is characterized by immune cell infiltration into target tissues to orchestrate the killing and removal of infected/damaged cells, and subsequently to promote tissue repair and regeneration. Chronic inflammation occurs when an acute response fails to resolve due to the continued presence of an inducer of inflammation and/or lack of normal immunoregulation. The excessive and persistent presence of cytotoxic immune cells and their mediators play important roles in the pathogenesis of human diseases, including alcoholic liver disease (ALD).

Several proinflammatory mediators that contribute to the development of ALD against a background of failed immunoregulation have been proposed, and their relative contributions to alcohol-mediated liver toxicity and inflammation will be discussed below.

CONTRIBUTORS TO ALCOHOL-RELATED INFLAMMATION

Microbial Products

The vast number of bacteria (greater than the sum of our own body cells by perhaps an order of magnitude) and other microbes in the digestive system, and their impact on physiology and pathophysiology are only now being fully appreciated. Different bacterial phyla are stimulated (metabolizers of ethanol) or inhibited by alcohol in the gut [1]. The severity of ALD correlates with plasma levels of bacterial products in both human subjects [2-4], and experimental ALD [5-7]. Ethanol administration disrupts the gut epithelial barrier, resulting in increased translocation of bacteria from the gastrointestinal tract [8-10]. In addition, alcohol administration downregulates the expression of several intestinal antimicrobial molecules, resulting in bacterial overgrowth and enteric dysbiosis [11].

The immune system recognizes a wide range of bacterial products (otherwise known as 'pathogen associated molecular patterns,' or PAMPs), and one of the first identified and best understood is lipopolysaccharide (LPS), which plays a key role in ALD. Following translocation across the intestinal epithelium, LPS enters the circulation and is subsequently cleared by the liver, primarily through Kupffer cells and hepatocytes [12]. LPS binds its receptor Toll-like receptor 4 (TLR4) on these cells and triggers well-defined signaling cascades resulting in the production of inflammatory cytokines, which drive the recruitment of other inflammatory cells, thereby expanding the inflammatory environment [13]. Consequently, the liver bears the brunt of inflammation induced by gut-derived LPS. In addition to causing liver injury, LPS and its associated inflammation plays a pathological role in the later stages of ALD via its ability to activate hepatic stellate cells (HSCs), leading to fibrosis [14, 15]. Finally, hepatocyte injury due to excessive alcohol intake elevates the expression of liver TLR4, potentially perpetuating a vicious cycle of inflammation [16].

Pretreatment with antibiotics or probiotics mitigates the effect of alcohol on liver injury and improves liver function [17-19], and genetic ablation of TLR4 or its co-receptor Cluster of differentiation receptor 14 (CD14) reduces liver pathology and inflammation in response to alcoholic liver injury [20, 21].

In addition to Gram-negative bacteria that produce LPS, the gut houses a variety of microorganisms and viruses that can similarly leak to the liver following alcohol exposure, and promote inflammation.

Co-infections with opportunistic pathogens (which can include otherwise commensal organisms in the healthy individual) or obligate pathogens, most notably the hepatitis viruses, typically exacerbate damage due to chronic alcohol intake. This is at least partly driven by the inflammation such infections induce, as described further below.

Alcohol Metabolites and Reactive Oxygen Species

Alcohol itself is inherently a direct immunotoxic substance. Furthermore, the ethanol metabolites acetaldehyde and acetate can directly induce inflammatory signaling in Kupffer cells/macrophages [22], and potentiate LPS-mediated induction of proinflammatory cytokines [23]. In addition, acetate is a substrate for mitochondrial energy production via the tricarboxylic acid cycle, which leads to increased reactive oxygen species (ROS) production. As well as causing direct hepatocyte injury, ROS amplify inflammatory signaling, and can also induce liver fibrosis. Underlining the important role of ROS in mediating ethanol damage, treatment with antioxidants and deletion of the p47phox subunit of NADPH oxidase in ethanol-fed animals reduced oxidative stress, inflammation and prevented liver injury [24, 25].

Perpetuating the Inflammatory Environment: Fatty Acids, Damaged Cells, and Hepatitis Viruses

Alcohol-induced liver steatosis is defined by accumulation of fatty acids in the liver. Apart from direct liver cell damage, saturated fatty acids (SFAs) perpetuate the inflammatory environment by acting as ligands for TLR4 [26] on Kupffer cells, macrophages and hepatocytes. Additionally, SFAs can directly activate the inflammasome in hepatocytes, or stimulate hepatocytes to produce danger signals that activate the inflammasome in immune cells, thereby driving inflammation [27].

Another hallmark of ALD is hepatocyte necrosis, which can be induced by activated neutrophils (see below), alcohol-related oxidative stress and pro-inflammatory cytokine signaling [28]. These necrotic cells can also activate the phagocytic cell inflammasome [29], as well as releasing RNA and DNA, which induce inflammation via TLR7/9 [30].

Along with necrosis, apoptosis is also a prominent feature of ALD [28]. Apoptotic cells activate the classical complement pathway in the liver via C1q [31]. Deletion of C1q abolishes ethanol-induced complement activation, and reduces ethanol-induced liver injury.

Finally, alcohol consumption in patients with hepatitis virus infection, particularly hepatitis C virus (HCV) infection, can accelerate the process of ALD. In immunocompetent HCV^+ subjects without alcoholism, chronic active hepatitis, cirrhosis, and hepatocellular carcinoma (HCC) develop at ~10, 21, and 29 years post-infection, respectively. Alcoholism increases these rates substantially. HCV triggers dysfunction and apoptosis of lymphocytes, including T, NK and NKT cells, via NADPH oxidase-derived oxygen radicals, which might be enhanced by alcohol ROS production, subsequently accelerating liver fibrosis. Furthermore, HCV core and nonstructural proteins induce TLR4 expression in hepatocytes, and lead to enhanced the production of extracellular matrix by HSCs [32].

IMMUNE CELLS IN ALCOHOLIC LIVER DISEASE

Kupffer Cells

Resident phagocytic Kupffer cells (and infiltrating macrophages) play a complex role in the pathogenesis of ALD. As described above, when the liver is injured during the onset of ALD, Kupffer cells elicit immune and inflammatory responses by producing factors such as TNFα, TGFβ, and ROS [33].

TNFα was one of the first proinflammatory cytokines linked with ALD. Elevated circulating levels of TNFα are induced early in ALD, and are closely coupled to liver injury, being elevated in patients with alcoholic hepatitis, but not in alcoholics without liver disease. Genetic ablation of the TNFα receptor in rodents, or blockade with a TNFα neutralizing antibody reduces ALD [34]. However, the results of studies using TNFα antagonists used to treat patients with alcoholic hepatitis have been mixed [35].

TNFα has the potential to increase expression of SREBP-1c in the liver, a transcription factor that regulates fat synthesis, leading to alcoholic steatosis [36]. TGFβ on the other hand, plays a crucial role in the transdifferentiation of hepatic stellate cells into activated myoblastic cells, stimulating their production of extracellular matrix, leading to fibrosis and eventual cirrhosis [37].

However, Kupffer cells/infiltrating macrophages can also function in a host-protective role, as they remove damaged cells, play an important role in fibrolysis resolution, and produce hepatoprotective cytokines such as IL-6 [38]. IL-6 knockout mice have increased liver steatosis, ROS and hepatocyte apoptosis in response to alcohol feeding, which was preventable by administration of IL-6 [39].

Neutrophils

A defining feature of ALD is phagocytic neutrophil infiltration, controlled by IL-8 and IL-17, which are consistently elevated in the circulation of alcoholic patients [40]. The extent of neutrophil infiltrate positively correlates with level of hepatocyte injury, and following alcohol abstinence, the grade of neutrophil infiltrate declines, followed by increased monocyte infiltration and eventual resolution of inflammation.

Although neutrophil infiltrate may play a protective role for the host by killing and removing alcohol-damaged hepatocytes, their activation also contributes to the pathogenesis of hepatocellular damage through their release of ROS and proteases during oxidative burst [41].

Natural Killer (NK) and NKT Cells

The liver contains a unique complement of immune cells related to its frontline role in resistance to infections derived from the gut as well as parenteral infections such as malaria. The liver is specifically highly enriched in innate immune cells including phagocytic cells as above and both NK and NKT cells, considered to be innate lymphocytes [42, 43].

The major liver-resident populations of NK and NKT cells can have a protective role in ALD, blocking the activation of hepatic stellate cells and fibrosis. Both cell types can directly kill activated but not quiescent hepatic stellate cells. They also produce interferon γ (IFNγ), which induces HSC cell cycle arrest and apoptosis [32].

However, the anti-fibrotic effects of NKT cells are only beneficial in the early stages of ALD; strong activation of iNKT with a single injection of their ligand α-galactosylceramide after disease is established, adversely enhanced liver fibrosis via increased IFNγ-mediated hepatocyte apoptosis [44]. Chronic stimulation of human NKT cells by increased hepatic expression of CD1d, specifically in chronic hepatitis C, appears to contribute to fibrosis and cirrhosis [45, 46]. Interestingly, however, alcoholics with hepatitis C down-regulate hepatic CD1d [46], although other direct pro-fibrotic mechanisms may then kick in, given the accelerated nature of chronic hepatitis C in the context of continued alcohol use.

It is also now believed that chronic alcohol consumption accelerates liver fibrosis partly because of the suppressed activities of NK cells. In patients with alcoholic liver cirrhosis, the number and cytolytic activity of NK cells are significantly decreased compared to those of patients without liver disease. However, it is not clear whether reduction of NK number is a cause or effect of ALD [32].

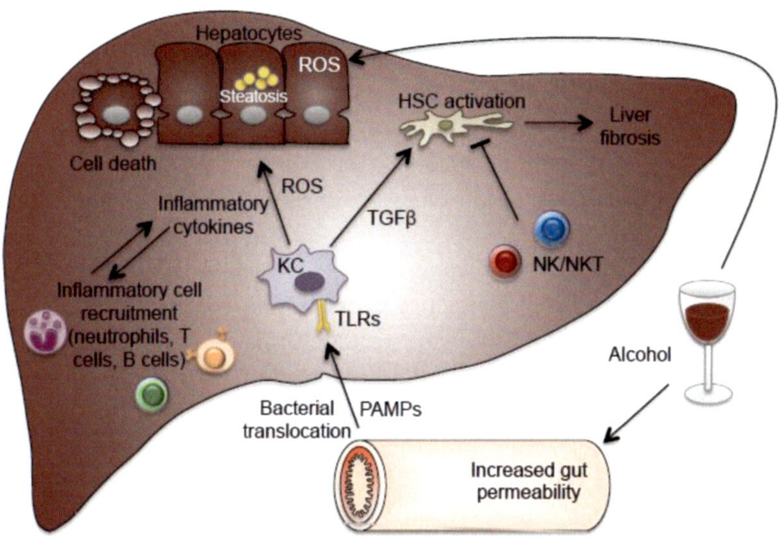

Figure 1. Inflammation in alcoholic liver disease. Alcohol alone (or its metabolites) increase intestinal permeability leading to increased bacterial and endotoxin translocation to the liver via the portal circulatory system. Activation of Kupffer cells through TLR recognition of PAMPs leads to increased production of inflammatory cytokines and ROS, resulting in hepatocyte injury and activation of HSCs. In addition, alcohol can directly induce inflammatory ROS production by hepatocytes and KCs. Liver resident NK and NKT cells can have a protective role in ALD, blocking the activation of HSCs and fibrosis. Increased liver inflammation drives the recruitment of inflammatory cells including neutrophils, T cells and B cells, thereby expanding the inflammatory environment and perpetuating liver inflammation.

T and B Lymphocytes

The activation of adaptive immunity during ALD is not as well defined as the innate. However potential activators include adducts generated by the reaction of ethanol metabolite acetaldehyde with proteins/lipids. These are commonly observed in alcohol-fed animals and alcoholic subjects [47]. As well as stimulating inflammatory responses in Kupffer cells, they have also been shown to activate cytotoxic T cells and induce adduct-specific antibody production [48].

Finally, while chronic high-level alcohol consumption is clearly hepatotoxic, abstinence prior to end-stage cirrhosis can have remarkable benefits due to the regenerative nature of the liver, resulting also in relative normalization of immune populations in the liver. Furthermore, direct injection of alcohol into liver tumours can have therapeutic effects [49].

CONCLUSION

In summary, the immune system contributes to ALD through chronic inflammation (Figure 1). However, immune components can also be protective, and restoring the balance of the healthy hepatic immune system promises to contribute to restoration of health in ALD. Therefore, when developing effective anti-inflammatory interventions, the challenge remains to identify the components and pathways that are primarily pathogenic and/or to develop strategies that mitigate the pathogenic effect without significantly compromising the protective functions of these components.

REFERENCES

[1] Zhong, W., Zhou, Z. Alterations of the gut microbiome and metabolome in alcoholic liver disease. *World journal of gastrointestinal pathophysiology*. 2014;5(4):514-22.

[2] Lin, R. S., Lee, F. Y., Lee, S. D., Tsai, Y. T., Lin, H. C., Lu, R. H. et al. Endotoxemia in patients with chronic liver diseases: relationship to severity of liver diseases, presence of esophageal varices, and hyperdynamic circulation. *Journal of hepatology*. 1995;22 (2):165-72.

[3] Fukui, H., Brauner, B., Bode, J. C., Bode, C. Plasma endotoxin concentrations in patients with alcoholic and non-alcoholic liver disease: reevaluation with an improved chromogenic assay. *Journal of hepatology*. 1991;12(2):162-9.

[4] Schafer, C., Parlesak, A., Schutt, C., Bode, J. C., Bode, C. Concentrations of lipopolysaccharide-binding protein, bactericidal/ permeability-increasing protein, soluble CD14 and plasma lipids in relation to endotoxaemia in patients with alcoholic liver disease. *Alcohol and alcoholism*. 2002;37(1):81-6.

[5] Tabata, T., Tani, T., Endo, Y., Hanasawa, K. Bacterial translocation and peptidoglycan translocation by acute ethanol administration. *Journal of gastroenterology*. 2002;37(9): 726-31.

[6] Guarner, C., Gonzalez-Navajas, J. M., Sanchez, E., Soriando, G., Frances, R., Chiva, M. et al. The detection of bacterial DNA in blood of rats with CCl4-induced cirrhosis with ascites represents episodes of bacterial translocation. *Hepatology*. 2006;44(3):633-9.

[7] Tamai, H., Kato, S., Horie, Y., Ohki, E., Yokoyama, H., Ishii, H. Effect of acute ethanol administration on the intestinal absorption of endotoxin in rats. *Alcoholism, clinical and experimental research*. 2000;24(3):390-4.

[8] Basuroy, S., Sheth, P., Mansbach, C. M., Rao, R. K. Acetaldehyde disrupts tight junctions and adherens junctions in human colonic mucosa: protection by EGF and L-glutamine. *American journal of physiology Gastrointestinal and liver physiology*. 2005; 289(2):G367-75.

[9] Bode, C., Bode, J. C. Effect of alcohol consumption on the gut. *Best practice and research Clinical gastroenterology*. 2003;17(4):575-92.

[10] Ferrier, L., Berard, F., Debrauwer, L., Chabo, C., Langella, P., Bueno, L. et al. Impairment of the intestinal barrier by ethanol involves enteric microflora and mast cell activation in rodents. *The American journal of pathology*. 2006;168(4):1148-54.

[11] Yan, A. W., Fouts, D. E., Brandl, J., Starkel, P., Torralba, M., Schott, E. et al. Enteric dysbiosis associated with a mouse model of alcoholic liver disease. *Hepatology*. 2011; 53(1):96-105.

[12] Wang, H. J., Zakhari, S., Jung, M. K. Alcohol, inflammation, and gut-liver-brain interactions in tissue damage and disease development. *World journal of gastroenterology: WJG*. 2010;16(11):1304-13.

[13] Mandrekar, P., Szabo, G. Signalling pathways in alcohol-induced liver inflammation. *Journal of hepatology*. 2009;50(6):1258-66.

[14] Csak, T., Velayudham, A., Hritz, I., Petrasek, J., Levin, I., Lippai, D. et al. Deficiency in myeloid differentiation factor-2 and toll-like receptor 4 expression attenuates nonalcoholic steatohepatitis and fibrosis in mice. *American journal of physiology Gastrointestinal and liver physiology*. 2011;300(3):G433-41.

[15] Seki, E., De Minicis, S., Osterreicher, C. H., Kluwe, J., Osawa, Y., Brenner, D. A. et al. TLR4 enhances TGF-beta signaling and hepatic fibrosis. *Nature medicine*. 2007;13(11): 1324-32.

[16] Gustot, T., Lemmers, A., Moreno, C., Nagy, N., Quertinmont, E., Nicaise, C. et al. Differential liver sensitization to toll-like receptor pathways in mice with alcoholic fatty liver. *Hepatology*. 2006;43(5):989-1000.

[17] Adachi, Y., Moore, L. E., Bradford, B. U., Gao, W., Thurman, R. G. Antibiotics prevent liver injury in rats following long-term exposure to ethanol. *Gastroenterology*. 1995;108(1):218-24.

[18] Kirpich, I. A., Solovieva, N. V., Leikhter, S. N., Shidakova, N. A., Lebedeva, O. V., Sidorov, P. I. et al. Probiotics restore bowel flora and improve liver enzymes in human alcohol-induced liver injury: a pilot study. *Alcohol*. 2008;42(8):675-82.

[19] Nanji, A. A., Khettry, U., Sadrzadeh, S. M. Lactobacillus feeding reduces endotoxemia and severity of experimental alcoholic liver (disease). *Proceedings of the Society for Experimental Biology and Medicine Society for Experimental Biology and Medicine*. 1994;205(3):243-7.

[20] Yin, M., Bradford, B. U., Wheeler, M. D., Uesugi, T., Froh, M., Goyert, S. M. et al. Reduced early alcohol-induced liver injury in CD14-deficient mice. *Journal of immunology*. 2001;166(7):4737-42.

[21] Hritz, I., Mandrekar, P., Velayudham, A., Catalano, D., Dolganiuc, A., Kodys, K. et al. The critical role of toll-like receptor (TLR) 4 in alcoholic liver disease is independent of the common TLR adapter MyD88. *Hepatology*. 2008;48(4):1224-31.

[22] Shen, Z., Ajmo, J. M., Rogers, C. Q., Liang, X., Le, L., Murr, M. M. et al. Role of SIRT1 in regulation of LPS- or two ethanol metabolites-induced TNF-alpha production in cultured macrophage cell lines. *American journal of physiology Gastrointestinal and liver physiology*. 2009;296(5):G1047-53.

[23] Enomoto, N., Schemmer, P., Ikejima, K., Takei, Y., Sato, N., Brenner, D. A. et al. Long-term alcohol exposure changes sensitivity of rat

Kupffer cells to lipopolysaccharide. *Alcoholism, clinical and experimental research.* 2001;25(9):1360-7.

[24] Kono, H., Rusyn, I., Yin, M., Gabele, E., Yamashina, S., Dikalova, A. et al. NADPH oxidase-derived free radicals are key oxidants in alcohol-induced liver disease. *The Journal of clinical investigation.* 2000;106(7):867-72.

[25] Wheeler, M. D., Kono, H., Yin, M., Rusyn, I., Froh, M., Connor, H. D. et al. Delivery of the Cu/Zn-superoxide dismutase gene with adenovirus reduces early alcohol-induced liver injury in rats. *Gastroenterology.* 2001;120(5):1241-50.

[26] Shi, H., Kokoeva, M. V., Inouye, K., Tzameli, I., Yin, H., Flier, J. S. TLR4 links innate immunity and fatty acid-induced insulin resistance. *The Journal of clinical investigation.* 2006;116(11):3015-25.

[27] Csak, T., Ganz, M., Pespisa, J., Kodys, K., Dolganiuc, A., Szabo, G. Fatty acid and endotoxin activate inflammasomes in mouse hepatocytes that release danger signals to stimulate immune cells. *Hepatology.* 2011;54(1):133-44.

[28] Nanji, A. A., Hiller-Sturmhofel, S. Apoptosis and necrosis: two types of cell death in alcoholic liver disease. *Alcohol health and research world.* 1997;21(4):325-30.

[29] Iyer, S. S., Pulskens, W. P., Sadler, J. J., Butter, L. M., Teske, G. J., Ulland, T. K. et al. Necrotic cells trigger a sterile inflammatory response through the Nlrp3 inflammasome. *Proceedings of the National Academy of Sciences of the United States of America.* 2009;106(48):20388-93.

[30] Imaeda, A. B., Watanabe, A., Sohail, M. A., Mahmood, S., Mohamadnejad, M., Sutterwala, F. S. et al. Acetaminophen-induced hepatotoxicity in mice is dependent on Tlr9 and the Nalp3 inflammasome. *The Journal of clinical investigation.* 2009;119(2): 305-14.

[31] Cohen, J. I., Roychowdhury, S., McMullen, M. R., Stavitsky, A. B., Nagy, L. E. Complement and alcoholic liver disease: role of C1q in the pathogenesis of ethanol-induced liver injury in mice. *Gastroenterology.* 2010;139(2):664-74, 74 e1.

[32] Suh, Y. G., Jeong, W. I. Hepatic stellate cells and innate immunity in alcoholic liver disease. *World journal of gastroenterology: WJG.* 2011;17(20):2543-51.

[33] Dixon, L. J., Barnes, M., Tang, H., Pritchard, M. T., Nagy, L. E. Kupffer cells in the liver. *Comprehensive Physiology.* 2013;3(2):785-97.

[34] Yin, M., Wheeler, M. D., Kono, H., Bradford, B. U., Gallucci, R. M., Luster, M. I. et al. Essential role of tumor necrosis factor alpha in alcohol-induced liver injury in mice. *Gastroenterology*. 1999;117(4):942-52.

[35] Frazier, T. H., Stocker, A. M., Kershner, N. A., Marsano, L. S., McClain, C. J. Treatment of alcoholic liver disease. *Therapeutic advances in gastroenterology*. 2011;4 (1):63-81.

[36] Endo, M., Masaki, T., Seike, M., Yoshimatsu, H. TNF-alpha induces hepatic steatosis in mice by enhancing gene expression of sterol regulatory element binding protein-1c (SREBP-1c). *Experimental biology and medicine*. 2007;232(5):614-21.

[37] Gressner, A. M. Transdifferentiation of hepatic stellate cells (Ito cells) to myofibroblasts: a key event in hepatic fibrogenesis. *Kidney international Supplement*. 1996;54:S39-45.

[38] Duffield, J. S., Forbes, S. J., Constandinou, C. M., Clay, S., Partolina, M., Vuthoori, S. et al. Selective depletion of macrophages reveals distinct, opposing roles during liver injury and repair. *The Journal of clinical investigation*. 2005;115(1):56-65.

[39] El-Assal, O., Hong, F., Kim, W. H., Radaeva, S., Gao, B. IL-6-deficient mice are susceptible to ethanol-induced hepatic steatosis: IL-6 protects against ethanol-induced oxidative stress and mitochondrial permeability transition in the liver. *Cellular and molecular immunology*. 2004;1(3):205-11.

[40] Xu, R., Huang, H., Zhang, Z., Wang, F. S. The role of neutrophils in the development of liver diseases. *Cellular and molecular immunology*. 2014;11(3):224-31.

[41] Ramaiah, S. K., Jaeschke, H. Hepatic neutrophil infiltration in the pathogenesis of alcohol-induced liver injury. *Toxicology mechanisms and methods*. 2007;17(7):431-40.

[42] Exley, M. A., Koziel, M. J. To be or not to be NKT: natural killer T cells in the liver. *Hepatology*. 2004;40(5):1033-40.

[43] Crispe, I. N. Liver antigen-presenting cells. *Journal of hepatology*. 2011; 54(2):357-65.

[44] Park, O., Jeong, W. I., Wang, L., Wang, H., Lian, Z. X., Gershwin, M. E. et al. Diverse roles of invariant natural killer T cells in liver injury and fibrosis induced by carbon tetrachloride. *Hepatology*. 2009;49(5):1683-94.

[45] Durante-Mangoni, E., Wang, R., Shaulov, A., He, Q., Nasser, I., Afdhal, N. et al. Hepatic CD1d expression in hepatitis C virus infection and

recognition by resident proinflammatory CD1d-reactive T cells. *Journal of immunology*. 2004;173(3):2159-66.

[46] Yanagisawa, K., Yue, S., van der Vliet, H. J., Wang, R., Alatrakchi, N., Golden-Mason, L. et al. Ex vivo analysis of resident hepatic pro-inflammatory CD1d-reactive T cells and hepatocyte surface CD1d expression in hepatitis C. *Journal of viral hepatitis*. 2013; 20(8):556-65.

[47] Mathews S, Feng D, Maricic I, Ju C, Kumar V, Gao B. Invariant natural killer T cells contribute to chronic-plus-binge ethanol-mediated liver injury by promoting hepatic neutrophil infiltration. Cell Mol Immunol. 2015 Feb 9. doi: 10.1038/cmi.2015.06. [Epub]

[48] Tuma, D. J., Thiele, G. M., Xu, D., Klassen, L. W., Sorrell, M. F. Acetaldehyde and malondialdehyde react together to generate distinct protein adducts in the liver during long-term ethanol administration. *Hepatology*. 1996;23(4):872-80.

[49] Viitala, K., Israel, Y., Blake, J. E., Niemela, O. Serum IgA, IgG, and IgM antibodies directed against acetaldehyde-derived epitopes: relationship to liver disease severity and alcohol consumption. *Hepatology*. 1997;25(6):1418-24.

[50] Jansen, M. C., van Hillegersberg, R., Chamuleau, R. A., van Delden, O. M., Gouma, D. J., van Gulik, T. M. Outcome of regional and local ablative therapies for hepatocellular carcinoma: a collective review. *European journal of surgical oncology: the journal of the European Society of Surgical Oncology and the British Association of Surgical Oncology*. 2005;31(4):331-47.

ion of miR-155, but not miR-125b, occurs after a macrophage cell line
264.7) is exposed to a prolonged alcohol treatment [19, 20]. Indeed,
macrophages exposed to alcohol or miR-155 overexpression show
ed sensitivity to LPS and higher TNF-α production, when compared to
ed control cells and such sensitization can be completely blocked by an
R-155 inhibitor. In addition, increased levels of miR-155 and TNF-α
ion were also found in isolated KCs from a mouse model of alcoholic
sease as compared with pair-fed controls. Altogether, these findings
a role for miR-155 overexpression in sensitized alcohol-exposed KCs
stimulation, thus amplifying inflammation induction. In this regard,
g miR-155 to inhibit TNF-α formation in KCs, without impairing the
nmune system, may prove beneficial in ALD patients.

PURINERGIC SIGNALING

ochondria generate intracellular ATP, which serves as the fundamental
currency on which life depends. However, when ATP or derivatives
ased into the extracellular milieu, as following trauma or cellular
, these metabolites act as danger molecules or DAMPs.
acellular ATP signals through type-2 purinergic receptor (P2R) e.g.,
eceptors, modulate inflammation in an inflammasome-dependent
Ectonucleotidases scavenge ATP to terminate these danger signals,
y generating adenosine. Interestingly, the derivative nucleosides have
rotective, anti-inflammatory and/or immunosuppressive properties,
e mediated *via* type-1 purinergic receptor e.g., A_{2A} (Figure 1).
have shown that CD39 expression by the vasculature and on innate
tive immune cells has protective properties in models of inflammation
is. This ectonucleotidase is most abundant in the immune system and
ilature with its expression modulated by inflammatory stress and/or
reactions. During inflammation, there is early functional loss of
s a consequence of oxidative stress. There is then constitutive
ion of CD39, which is provoked by hypoxia, cytokines (IL-6 and IL-
ryl hydrocarbon receptor activation, as with unconjugated bilirubin.

In: Alcohol and the Liver
Editor: Gerond Lake-Bakaar
ISBN: 978-1-63484-400-0

Chapter 3

PURINERGIC SIGNALING AND THE INFLAMMASOME IN ACUTE ALCOHOLIC LIVER DISEASE

Paola de Adrade Mello[1,2], Trishan Vaikunthanathan[3] and Simon C. Robson[2,*]

[1]Faculty of Pharmacy, Federal University of Rio Grande do Sul, Porto Alegre, Rio Grande do Sul, Brazil
[2]Division of Gastroenterology BIDMC, Harvard Medical School, Boston, MA, US
[3]MRC Centre for Transplantation, Division of Transplantation Immunology & Mucosal Biology King's College London, London, UK

ABSTRACT

Alcoholic liver disease (ALD) comprises a range of disorders including alcoholic fatty liver (steatosis), alcoholic steatohepatitis with or without fibrosis, cirrhosis and hepatocellular cancer. Acute alcoholic hepatitis is the most severe form of the disease with high mortality and limited treatment options. Liver inflammation is the main characteristic of acute hepatitis and plays a central role in ALD progression.

* Corresponding author: Simon C. robson. Division of Gastroenterology BIDMC, Harvard Medical School, Boston, MA, US. E-mail: srobson@bidmc.harvard.edu.

Understanding ALD pathogenesis in the context of inflammation and hepatocellular dysfunction may provide new insights for the disease treatment as well as facilitate discovery of novel targets to control disease progression.

In this chapter, we highlight aspects of purinergic signaling and inflammasome activation as important components of hepatic pathophysiology in ALD. Inflammasomes are intracellular multiprotein complexes that mediate cellular response to exogenous and endogenous danger signals resulting in immune cell activation and recruitment. When activated by extracellular nucleotides e.g., ATP *via* type 2 purinergic receptors, by derivative nucleosides such as adenosine or penultimate metabolites uric acid, the inflammasome promotes capase-1 activation resulting in IL-1β and IL-18 maturation and release. Patients with ALD exhibit high levels of IL-1β, noted also in models of alcoholic hepatitis. Consequently there are links to inflammasome activation in ALD onset and progression. We review the studies that link inflammasome activation to manifestations of disease, such as steatosis, liver inflammation and fibrosis, in ALD. Precise mechanisms involved in ALD still need to be elucidated and therapeutic options explored.

INTRODUCTION

Alcoholic liver disease (ALD) is one of the leading causes of mortality in the United States, claiming over 12,000 lives each year [1, 2]. The scale of injury in ALD is described along a disease spectrum ranging through alcoholic fatty liver (steatosis) and alcoholic steatohepatitis (ASH) with or without fibrosis to cirrhosis and hepatocellular cancer, the latter two necessitating transplantation [3]. While steatosis and the early phases of steatohepatitis are reversible following the cessation of alcohol abuse [3], acute ASH is considered the most severe form of the disease contributing heavily to ALD-related mortality[4].

Despite the high mortality and ever-growing prevalence of ALD, there is still no definitive therapy to treat or prevent its progression, partly substantiated by a relative paucity of research in the field. As such, a better understanding of the pathogenic mechanisms underlying this disease might bring to light new perspectives in ALD treatment, directing the discovery of novel targeted therapies and addressing a clinically unmet need.

In this chapter, we address and briefly discuss the importance of inflammation and purinergic signaling in acute ALD pathogenesis highlighting

the role of the inflammasome in the manisfestation disease.

UNDERSTANDING INFLAMMA ELEMENTS OF ALD PATHOG

We generally accept that liver inflammation anc innate immune system is associated with disease Additionally, other factors such as toxic products fr oxidative stress, acetaldehyde adducts, abnormal malnutrition, the activation of systemic immunity by enter *via* "leaky" mucosal barriers in the gut, regeneration are also relevant and must be considered

Liver inflammation is associated with exposure exogenous and endogenous triggers [6]. The most co of liver inflammation is the gut-derived (lipopolysaccharide; LPS). Alcohol metabolism in production of toxic metabolites which disrupt the int increasing membrane permeability, and in turn prom LPS to the portal circulation[7]. On the other hand, t sterile, triggers has not been fully clarified, but a rol signals, such as uric acid and ATP has been proposed

The exogenous trigger LPS is recognized by liv Kupffer Cells (KC) through Toll like receptor 4 (T activation and induction of proinflammatory cytoki IL-8 and TNF-α [9, 10]. TNF-α is increased in immunohistochemical staining in patients with previous studies have pointed a role for this cytokin ALD [11-14]. However, human clinical trials usir were discontinued on account of its poor side-effe were found to be more susceptible to infection [15, 1

TNF-α production can also be modulated by mic role for miR-155 and miR-125b has already been de miR-155 enhances TNF-α translation and miR transcriptional repressor of TNF-α. In macroph induction involves TLR4 and NFk-B activation [1 increased production of TNF-α. Previous work has s

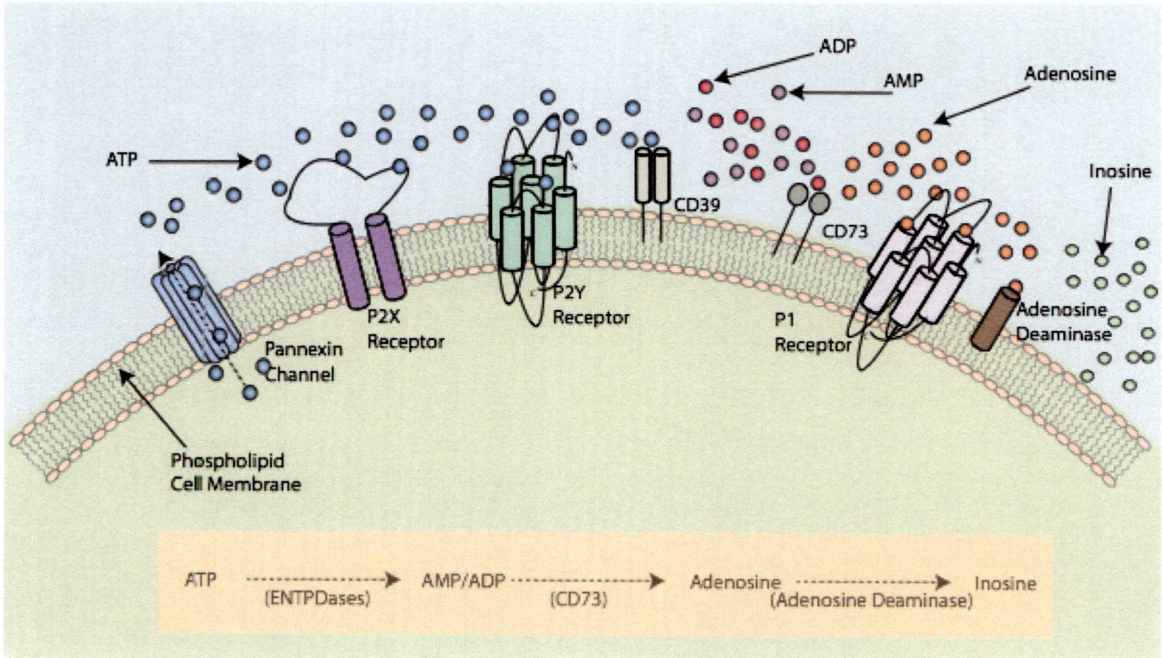

Figure 1. An Overview of Purinergic Signaling. Intracellular ATP is released from cells through the opening of pannexin hemi channels, where it can serve as an extracellular signaling molecule. ATP subsequently signals with various P2 receptors, both ligand-gated P2X and G protein coupled P2Y receptors, in an autocrine manner. This signaling process has been implicated in a wide variety of physiological processes. Eventually, ATP is hydrolysed by cell surface expressed ENTPDases, including CD39, and the ecto-5'-nucleotidase, CD73 which promotes the generation of adenosine. Adenosine signals on G-protein coupled P1 receptors and is metabolised to inosine by the enzyme adenine deaminase.

ATP and DAMPs may drive inflammation, such as that seen in ALD, *via* interactions with neutrophils. In this context, CD39 and CD73 on myeloid cells play a crucial role by controlling the extracellular ATP levels. We already know that impairment of nucleotide catabolism by pharmacologic inhibition or genetic deletion of CD39 or CD73 increases the activation, chemotaxis, and adhesion of neutrophils to the vascular endothelium [21-24].

P2X7R signaling on myeloid cells is pro-inflammatory. Importantly, eATP activates the NLRP3 inflammasome [25], leading to the maturation and release of IL-1β and IL-18 [26].

As an example of CD39-mediated suppression of inflammation, we have found that treatment with IL-27 drives CD39 expression and can suppress NLRP3 inflammasome activation in dendritic cells (DC) and decreases secretion of IL-1β. Furthermore, in concordance with this data,, the inhibitory effects of IL-27 on NLRP3 inflammasome activation and subsequent IL-1β release are negated in IL-27RA^{KO} or CD39^{KO} DCs.

Taken together, these data suggest that the upregulation of CD39 triggered by IL-27 decreases eATP levels and consequently, limits NLRP3 inflammasome activation. However, whereas extracellular nucleotides are accepted as danger molecules or DAMPS that activate the inflammasome, the derivative nucleosides are usually considered to be innate protective molecules, which are generally thought to have anti-inflammatory/ immunoregulatory properties [27]. Inflammatory cytokines are known to drive chronic diseases but we do not yet understand how sustained activation of myeloid cells can be maintained. Signals such as TLR agonists induce acute cytokine production by macrophages, but this is not sustained, and cells become unresponsive to additional stimuli [28].

Myeloid cells typically serve as the first line of defense in response to harmful endogenous or exogenous agents, such as invading pathogens, inducing the innate immune response. Since neutrophils are also able to migrate toward the inflammatory focus, as with liver injury, and trigger a series of pathogenetic effector mechanisms, these cells are also crucial effectors of the innate immunity.

Inflammatory mediators released from macrophages, such as chemokines and ATP, activate and promote neutrophil migration to the sites of inflammation [29]. Macrophage activation usually depends on Toll-like receptor (TLR) activation by pathogen-associated molecular patterns (PAMPs) or DAMPs. Upon TLR activation, macrophages release ATP inducing pro-inflammatory responses through the activation of P2 receptors, including leukocyte migration and activation [29, 30]. CD39/ENTPD1 is the major ectonucleotidase expressed by macrophages and plays an important immunomodulatory role by regulating the extracellular ATP levels and limiting P2-mediated cellular responses, such as apoptosis, NLRP3 inflammasome activation, and IL-β release [31]. Macrophages also co-express CD73, thus allowing for the production of adenosine.

The adenosine generated by the CD39/CD73 axis is crucial to limit macrophage responses acting via A_{2B} receptors [30]. Furthermore, ectonucleotidases are down regulated in pro-inflammatory M1 macrophages and upregulated in M2 macrophages, which are able to generate an adenosine-rich anti-inflammatory and pro-resolution environment [30, 32].

Uric acid is the major end product of purine catabolism and is pathologically released from injured cells, representing an endogenous danger signal that activates the NALP3/NLRP3 inflammasome and leads to IL-1 β production [33, 34]. At high local concentrations, uric acid precipitates and forms monosodium urate (MSU) crystals, which represents a potent inflammasome activator and drive tissue inflammation, as observed in clinical gout [35].

Purinergic Modulation of Inflammation and Immune Responses in ALD

TNF-α, IL-6, IL-8 and IL-1 are all increased in the serum of patients with ALD [12, 14, 36, 37]. The role of IL-6 in ALD is complex and not completely understood, but studies suggest protective effects in the early phase of this disease. IL-6 has been reported to protect hepatocyte apoptosis and participate in mitochondrial DNA repair after alcoholic liver injury [38, 39]. IL-8 is a crucial proinflammatory cytokine linked to neutrophil mobilization from bone marrow to the liver, but its significance in ALD still remains to be elucidated [40]. Amongst all these cytokines, data suggests that IL 1 plays the most critical role in ALD progression. Accordingly, IL-1 (IL-1β albeit not IL-1α) signaling is crucial in alcohol-induced steatosis, inflammation and hepatocyte damage [41].

IL-1β is a potent proinflamatory cytokine produced as inactive pro-IL-1β in response to inflammatory stimuli, such as microbial products (LPS for example) and endogenous danger-associated molecules (ATP and uric acid for example). IL-1β gene expression and synthesis of pro–IL-1β occurs after activation of pattern recognition receptors (PRRs), such as TLR4.

Inflammatory stimuli also lead to activation of cytosolic CARD and PYHIN domain–containing PRRs that recruit the adaptor ASC and caspase-1 (Casp-1) to assemble into the multiprotein complex inflammasome on cytosol. Pro–Casp-1 activated by the inflammasome, cleaves pro–IL-1β into the bioactive IL-1β [42]. After being released, IL-1β acts in an autocrine/paracrine way *via* the type I IL-1 receptor (IL-1R1). The interaction IL-1β/IL-1R1 is normally blocked by the naturally occurring IL-1 receptor antagonist (IL-1Ra), which inhibits the biological response to IL-1 [41]. In an alcoholic steatohepatitis mouse model, the increase IL-1β release was mediated exclusively by liver immune cells (KC) and was Casp-1-ASC-inflammasome activation dependent, culminating in inflammation, steatosis, liver damage, and fibrosis. Moreover, all these ALD symptoms were ameliorated by pharmacological use of IL-1Ra (Anakinra), suggesting the therapeutic utility of IL-1 receptor blockade in alcohol-induced liver disease [41].

As described above, IL-1β maturation and release requires inflammasome assembly and consists of 2-steps. In the 1st step, exogenous microbial-derived signal activates pro-IL-1β production, culminating in synthesis of inactive pro-IL-1β. In ALD this step is triggered by LPS derived from the gut binding to TLR4 on KCs and represents the first proinflammatory signal [43-47]. Deficiency in TLR4 blocks pro-IL-1β up-regulation in the liver of alcoholic-fed mice [48].

The pro-IL-1β cleavage to the active IL-1β form represents the second step, the end result of inflammasome activation by endogenous signals derived from host cells, namely danger signals [42]. The nature of this danger signal in ALD has not yet been identified, however, studies have suggested the role of uric acid and ATP, released from ethanol-damaged hepatocytes [6, 8]. This assumption came from the fact that uric acid and ATP levels were increased in the serum of human volunteers exposed to a single dose of ethanol or in the supernatant of primary human hepatocytes exposed to ethanol.

Moreover, uric acid and ATP seems to mediated a paracrine inflammatory cross-talk between damaged hepatocytes and immune cells, as these danger signals released by hepatocytes significantly increased the expression of LPS-inducible cytokines, such as IL-1β and TNF-α by immune cells [8].

Finally, a crucial role of NLRP3, a ligand-sensing component of the inflammasome, which recognizes uric acid and ATP, was demonstrated in this setting. Accordingly, deficiency of NLRP3, prevented the development of alcohol induced liver inflammation in mice fed a Lieber-DeCarli ethanol diet and significantly ameliorated liver damaged and steatosis [8].

The importance of uric acid and ATP as sterile danger signal that leads to inflammasome activation in ALD was confirmed recently [6]. In a mouse model of alcoholic steatohepatitis (ASH), uric acid depletion using mice overexpressing uricase or lack of ATP signaling by using ATP receptor P2X7-KO mice resulted in ASH attenuation and prevented inflamosome activation and subsequent IL-1β release. In the same way, pharmacological depletion of uric acid with allopurinol showed a significant protection from alcohol-stimulated inflammatory response, steatosis and liver damage. Complete protection was only achieved when mice were treated with probenecid, a drug that promotes both uric acid depletion and ATP-induced P2X7 signaling blockade. Altogether, these findings reinforce a role of uric acid and ATP as a second danger signal leading to inflammasome activation and IL-1β release and consequently highlight the prospects of targeting these molecules in the treatment of ASH.

Some recent studies from Dr. Wajahat Mehal and colleagues have been particularly illuminating. As previously mentioned, IL-1 production was initially thought to only involve two types of signals a signal 1 which is typically a TLR agonist, and a signal 2 which can be diverse but in relation to the activation of macrophages, including cholesterol crystals/uric acid or other signals [49]. However, it has been recently shown that adenosine is a key third signal, which results in sustained production of IL-1β, and this is dependent on the A2R as well as HIF-1α [50].

Although inflammasome activation seems to be a requisite to the alcohol-induced liver inflammation, the exact role in ALD pathogenesis remains controversial. Members of the NOD-like receptor (NLR) family form an inflammasome that is activated by pathogens and signals released through local tissue injury or death [51]. NLR family pyrin domain containing 3 (NLRP3) responds to ATP, pore-forming toxins and uric acid [35, 52, 53], while NLR family CARD domain containing protein 4 (NLRC4) detects pathogenic bacteria such as Salmonella enteric server typhimurium (Salmonella), Legionella pneumophila (Legionella) and Pseudomonas aeruginosa (Pseudomonas) [54-59]. Both proteins are responsible for controlling caspase-1 activation and thus leading to IL-1β release.

In this way, deletion of NLRP3 and NLRC4 in an alcohol-induced liver injury mice model is expected to prevent ALD development. However, mice deficient in NLRP3 protein (Nlrp3−/−) developed severe liver injury, high plasma ALT and IL-18 levels, and reduced IL-1β after being subjected to continuous alcohol diet. Similarly, NLRC4-deficient mice (Nlrc4−/−) had reduced IL-1β production when exposed to chronic alcohol consumption.

Together these data present an unexpected protective effect for NLRP3 and NLRC4 inflammasome in ALD progression [60]. Considering that previous studies have shown an opposite effect for NLPR3 [8], future studies will determine the exactly role of NLPR3 inflammasome in the ALD development.

Although the crosstalk between damaged hepatocytes and immune cells are essential to ALD pathogenesis, a role for hepatic stellate cells (HSC) in liver fibrosis must also be considered. HSC, much like immune cells, go through functional changes in response to tissue injury and death, but the mechanism involved in this process are still poorly understood [61].

A role for inflammasome in this context has already been described and its activity seems to be important to liver fibrosis development [62].

An *in vitro* study using LX-2 cells and primary mouse HSC demonstrated that inflammasome activation by monosodiumurate (MSU) crystals produced functional changes to cells, including inhibition of chemotaxis, induction of actin reorganization and enhanced collagen1 and TGF-α expression. Moreover, in mice lacking inflammasome components (NLRP3 or ASC) the development of experimental liver fibrosis was significantly reduced [62]. Therefore, the inflammasome can also regulate a variety of HSC functions and seems to be important for liver fibrosis development. In this regard, understanding inflammasome-mediated regulation of HSC may be useful to find a new strategy for reducing collagen deposition.

Purinergic Links to Hepatic Fibrosis

Liver fibrosis associated with ALD is typically associated with chronic inflammation and excessive reparative responses. Excessive collagen accumulation in the liver sinusoids and progressive extension can lead to portal hypertension and loss of hepatic architecture resulting in aberrant regeneration and cirrhosis. Advanced cirrhosis results in liver failure, often requiring liver transplantation and is also linked to the development of hepatocellular carcinoma.

Myofibroblasts, portal fibroblasts and hepatic stellate cells are linked to the abnormal matrix deposition in the diseased liver. Activation of the A_{2A} receptor induces expression of collagen by stellate cells [63] and inhibition or deletion of this signaling prevents experimental, ethanol-induced fibrosis in mice [64].

Adenosine-mediated effects are also dependent on A_{2B} activation as the receptor antagonist MRS1754 reduces liver fibrosis as well [65, 66]. CD73 ecto -5'-nucleotidase has been linked to hepatic fibrosis given the generation of extracellular adenosine [67]. However, participation of this ectonucleotidase in healing is multifaceted as knockdown of CD73 induces an increase in collagen I and augments cell migration in stellate cells [68].

Curiously, multiple studies suggest a protective role of coffee in progressive liver fibrosis, liver cancer and cirrhosis [69]. Mechanistic studies of late suggest that benefit may be mediated by A_{2A}, where caffeine may serve as a selective inhibitor on hepatic stellate cells.

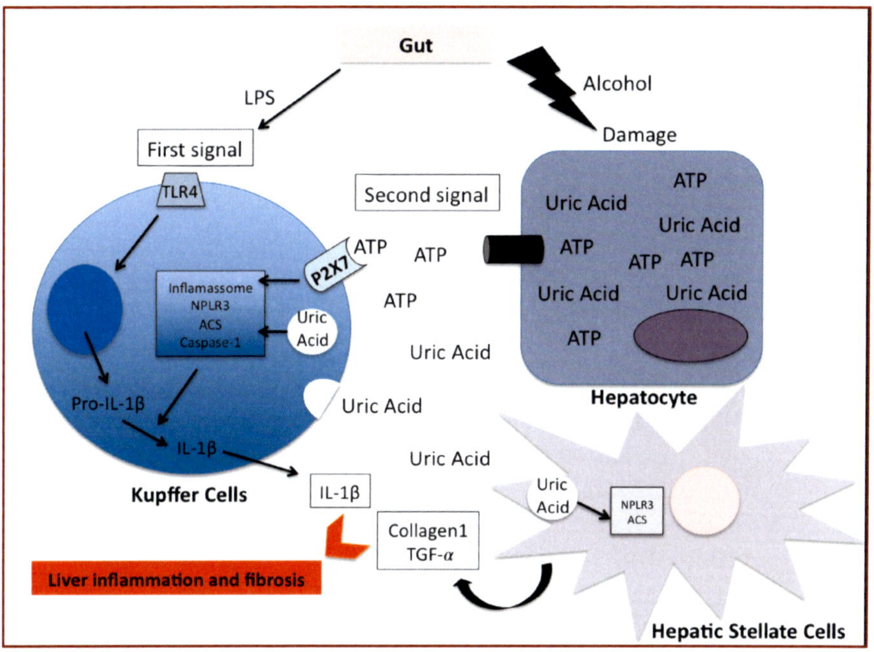

Figure 2. Schematic representation showing inflammasome involvement in ALD pathogenesis. Alcohol consumption leads to both hepatocyte damage and increase intestinal membrane permeability. While the later allows increase exposure of liver immune cells to LPS (first signal), the former augment the extracellular levels of ATP and uric acid (second signal), culminating in inflammasome activation and IL-1β release by liver immune cells (Kupffer Cells). Active IL-1β plays a crucial role in alcohol-induced liver inflammation. Besides immune cells, hepatic stellate cells (HSC) are also important to ALD pathogenesis. Exposing HSC to endogenous danger signals, such as ATP or uric acid, leads to inflammasome activation and collagen1 and TGF-α release, which promote liver fibrosis.

CONCLUSION

Despite several key advances in our understanding of the pathogenesis and clinical characteristics of ALD, many questions and clinical quandaries remain. At the present, therapeutic strategies to treat alcoholic hepatitis, based on corticosteroids administration, have limit benefit and carry the risk of infections [15, 16]. Therefore, discovering new agents that effectively treat ALD without side effects are urgently required. Here we discussed the potential involvement of inflammasome in acute alcoholic liver injury, with respects to its development and progression (Figure 2) and propose various strategies to manipulate purinergic signals as novel therapeutic targets in ALD.

REFERENCES

[1] Shaheen, N. J., Hansen, R. A., Morgan, D. R., Gangarosa, L. M., Ringel, Y., Thiny, M. T., Russo, M. W., Sandler, R. S. The burden of gastrointestinal and liver diseases. *Am. J. Gastroenterol.* 2006;101: 2128-2138.

[2] Rehm, J., Mathers, C., Popova, S., Thavorncharoensap, M., Teerawattananon, Y., Patra, J. Global burden of disease and injury and economic cost attributable to alcohol use and alcohol-use disorders. *Lancet.* 2009;373:2223-2233.

[3] O'Shea, R. S., Dasarathy, S., McCullough, A. J. Alcoholic liver disease. *Hepatology.* 2010;51(1):307-328.

[4] Szabo, G., Petrasek, J., Bala, S. Innate immunity and alcoholic liver disease. *Dig. Dis.* 2012;30(Suppl. 1):55-60.

[5] Haber, P. S., Warner, R., Seth, D., Gorrell, M. D., McCaughan, G. W. Pathogenesis and management of alcoholic hepatitis. *J. Gastroenterol. Hepatol.* 2003;18(12):1332-1344.

[6] Iracheta-Vellve, A., Petrasek, J., Satishchandran, A., Gyongyosi, B., Saha, B., Kodys, K., Fitzgerald, K. A., Kurt-Jones, E. A., Szabo, G. Inhibition of sterile danger signals, uric acid and ATP, prevents inflammasome activation and protects from alcoholic steatohepatitis in mice. *J. Hepatol.* 2015;63(5):1147-55.

[7] Rao, R. K., Seth, A., Sheth, P. Recent Advances in Alcoholic Liver Disease I. Role of intestinal permeability and endotoxemia in alcoholic

liver disease. *Am. J. Physiol. Gastrointest. Liver Physiol.* 2004; 286(6): G881-4.

[8] Petrasek, J., Iracheta-Vellve, A., Saha, B., Satishchandran, A., Kodys, K., Fitzgerald, K. A., Kurt-Jones, E. A., Szabo, G. Metabolic danger signals, uric acid and ATP, mediate inflammatory cross-talk between hepatocytes and immune cells in alcoholic liver disease. *J. Leukoc. Biol.* 2015;98(2):249-56.

[9] Fukui, H., Brauner, B., Bode, J. C., Bode, C. Plasma endotoxin concentrations in patients with alcoholic and non-alcoholic liver disease: reevaluation with an improved chromogenic assay. *J. Hepatol.* 1991;12 (2):162-169.

[10] Fujimoto, M., Uemura, M., Nakatani, Y. et al. Plasma endotoxin and serum cytokine levels in patients with alcoholic hepatitis: relation to severity of liver disturbance. *Alcohol. Clin. Exp. Res.* 2000;24(4): S48-S54.

[11] McClain, C., Hill, D., Schmidt, J., Diehl, A. M. Cytokines and alcoholic liver disease. *Semin. Liver Dis.* 1993;13:170-182.

[12] Iimuro, Y., Gallucci, R. M., Luster, M. I., Kono, H., Thurman, R. G. Antibodies to tumor necrosis factor alfa attenuate hepatic necrosis and inflammation caused by chronic exposure to ethanol in the rat. *Hepatology.* 1997;26:1530-1537.

[13] Thurman, R. G. II. Alcoholic liver injury involves activation of Kupffer cells by endotoxin. *Am. J. Physiol.* 1998;275:G605-G611.

[14] McClain, C. J., Barve, S., Barve, S., Deaciuc, I., Hill, D. B. Tumor necrosis factor and alcoholic liver disease. *Alcohol. Clin. Exp. Res.* 1998;22:248S-252S.

[15] Tilg, H., Jalan, R., Kaser, A., Davies, N. A., Offner, F. A., Hodges, S. J., Ludwiczek, O., Shawcross, D., Zoller, H., Alisa, A., Mookerjee, R. P., Graziadei, I., Datz, C., Trauner, M., Schuppan, D., Obrist, P., Vogel, W., Williams, R. Anti-tumor necrosis factor-alpha monoclonal antibody therapy in severe alcoholic hepatitis. *J. Hepatol.* 2003;38:419-425.

[16] Naveau, S., Chollet-Martin, S., Dharancy, S., Mathurin, P., Jouet, P., Piquet, M. A., Davion, T., Oberti, F., Broet, P., Emilie, D., Foie-Alcool group of the Association Francaise pour l'Etude du Foie. A double-blind randomized controlled trial of infliximab associated with prednisolone in acute alcoholic hepatitis. *Hepatology.* 2004;39:1390-1397.

[17] Tili, E., Michaille, J. J., Cimino, A., Costinean, S., Dumitru, C. D., Adair, B., Fabbri, M., Alder, H., Liu, C. G., Calin, G. A., Croce, C. M. Modulation of miR-155 and miR-125b levels following

lipopolysaccharide/TNF-alpha stimulation and their possible roles in regulating the response to endotoxin shock. *J. Immunol.* 2007;179:5082-5089.

[18] Taganov, K. D., Boldin, M. P., Chang, K. J., Baltimore, D. NF-kappaB-dependent induction of microRNA miR-146, an inhibitor targeted to signaling proteins of innate immune responses. *Proc. Natl. Acad. Sci. US.* 2006;103:12481-12486.

[19] Bala, S., Marcos, M., Kodys, K., Csak, T., Catalano, D., Mandrekar, P., Szabo, G. Up-regulation of microRNA-155 in macrophages contributes to increased tumor necrosis factor {alpha} (TNF{alpha}) production via increased mRNA half-life in alcoholic liver disease. *J. Biol. Chem.* 2011; 286:1436-1444.

[20] Bala, S., Marcos, M., Szabo, G. Emerging role of microRNAs in liver diseases. *World J. Gastroenterol.* 2009;15:5633-5640.

[21] Eltzschig, H. K., Thompson, L. F., Karhausen, J., Cotta, R. J., Ibla, J. C., Robson, S. C., Colgan, S. P. Endogenous adenosine produced during hypoxia attenuates neutrophil accumulation: coordination by extracellular nucleotide metabolism. *Blood.* 2004;104(13):3986-92.

[22] Corriden, R., Chen, Y., Inoue, Y., Beldi, G., Robson, S. C., Insel, P. A., Junger, W. G. Ecto-nucleoside triphosphate diphosphohydrolase 1 (E-NTPDase1/CD39) regulates neutrophil chemotaxis by hydrolyzing released ATP to adenosine. *J. Biol. Chem.* 2008;283(42):28480-6.

[23] Reutershan, J., Vollmer, I., Stark, S., Wagner, R., Ngamsri, K. C., Eltzschig, H. K. Adenosine and inflammation: CD39 and CD73 are critical mediators in LPS-induced PMN trafficking into the lungs. *FASEB J.* 2009;23(2):473-82.

[24] Kukulski, F., Bahrami, F., Ben Yebdri, F., Lecka, J., Martín-Satué, M., Lévesque, S. A., Sévigny, J. NTPDase1 controls IL-8 production by human neutrophils. *J. Immunol.* 2011;187(2):644-53.

[25] McDonald, B., Pittman, K., Menezes, G. B., Hirota, S. A., Slaba, I., Waterhouse, C. C., Beck, P. L., Muruve, D. A., Kubes, P. Intravascular danger signals guide neutrophils to sites of sterile inflammation. *Science.* 2010;330(6002):362-6.

[26] Gombault, A., Baron, L., Couillin, I. ATP release and purinergic signaling in NLRP3 inflammasome activation. *Front. Immunol.* 2013;3: 414.

[27] Eltzschig, H. K., Sitkovsky, M. V., Robson, S. C. Purinergic signaling during inflammation. *N. Engl. J. Med.* 2012;367(24):2322-33.

[28] Fleming, B. D., Mosser, D. M. Regulatory macrophages: setting the threshold for therapy. *Eur. J. Immunol.* 2011;41(9):2498-502.
[29] Kawamura, H., Kawamura, T., Kanda, Y., Kobayashi, T., Abo, T. Extracellular ATP-stimulated macrophages produce macrophage inflammatory protein-2 which is important for neutrophil migration. *Immunology.* 2012;136(4):448-58.
[30] Cohen, H. B., Briggs, K. T., Marino, J. P., Ravid, K., Robson, S. C., Mosser, D. M. TLR stimulation initiates a CD39-based autoregulatory mechanism that limits macrophage inflammatory responses. *Blood.* 2013;122(11):1935-45.
[31] Lévesque, S. A., Kukulski, F., Enjyoji, K., Robson, S. C., Sévigny, J. NTPDase1 governs P2X7-dependent functions in murine macrophages. *Eur. J. Immunol.* 2010;40(5):1473-85.
[32] Zanin, R. F., Braganhol, E., Bergamin, L. S., Campesato, L. F., Filho, A. Z., Moreira, J. C., Morrone, F. B., Sévigny, J., Schetinger, M. R., de Souza Wyse, A. T., Battastini, A. M. Differential macrophage activation alters the expression profile of NTPDase and ecto-5'-nucleotidase. *PLoS One.* 2012;7(2):e31205.
[33] Gasse, P., Riteau, N., Charron, S., Girre, S., Fick, L., Pétrilli, V., Tschopp, J., Lagente, V., Quesniaux, V. F., Ryffel, B., Couillin, I. Uric acid is a danger signal activating NALP3 inflammasome in lung injury inflammation and fibrosis. *Am. J. Respir. Crit. Care Med.* 2009 May 15; 179(10):903-13.
[34] Griffith, J. W., Sun, T., McIntosh, M. T., Bucala, R. Pure Hemozoin is inflammatory in vivo and activates the NALP3 inflammasome via release of uric acid. *J. Immunol.* 2009;183(8):5208-20.
[35] Martinon, F., Pétrilli, V., Mayor, A., Tardivel, A., Tschopp, J. Gout-associated uric acid crystals activate the NALP3 inflammasome. *Nature.* 2006;440(7081):237-41.
[36] Khoruts, A., Stauhnke, L., McClain, C. J., Logan, G., Allen, J. I. Circulating tumor necrosis factor, interleukin-1 and interleukin-6 concentrations in chronic alcoholic patients. *Hepatology.* 1991;13: 267-276.
[37] Miller, A. M., Horiguchi, N., Jeong, W. I., Radaeva, S., Gao, B. Molecular mechanisms of alcoholic liver disease: innate immunity and cytokines. *Alcohol. Clin. Exp. Res.* 2011;35:787-793.
[38] Sheron, N., Bird, G., Goka, J., Alexander, G., Williams, R. Elevated plasma interleukin-6 and increased severity and mortality in alcoholic hepatitis. *Clin. Exp. Immunol.* 1991;84(3):449-53.

[39] Hong, F., Kim, W. H., Tian, Z., Jaruga, B., Ishac, E., Shen, X., Gao, B. Elevated interleukin-6 during ethanol consumption acts as a potential endogenous protective cytokine against ethanol-induced apoptosis in the liver: involvement of induction of Bcl-2 and Bcl-xL proteins. *Oncogene.* 2002;21(1):32-43.

[40] Kawaratani, H., Tsujimoto, T., Douhara, A., Takaya, H., Moriya, K., Namisaki, T., Noguchi, R., Yoshiji, H., Fujimoto, M., Fukui, H. The effect of inflammatory cytokines in alcoholic liver disease. *Mediators Inflamm.* 2013;2013:495156.

[41] Petrasek, J., Bala, S., Csak, T., Lippai, D., Kodys, K., Menashy, V., Barrieau, M., Min, S. Y., Kurt-Jones, E. A., Szabo, G. IL-1 receptor antagonist ameliorates inflammasome-dependent alcoholic steatohepatitis in mice. *J. Clin. Invest.* 2012;122(10):3476-89.

[42] Schroder, K., Tschopp, J. The inflammasomes. *Cell.* 2010;140(6):821-832.

[43] Adachi, Y., Bradford, B. U., Gao, W., Bojes, H. K., Thurman, R. G. Inactivation of Kupffer cells prevents early alcohol-induced liver injury. *Hepatology.* 1994;20(2):453-60.

[44] Adachi, Y., Moore, L. E., Bradford, B. U., Gao, W., Thurman, R. G. Antibiotics prevent liver injury in rats following long-term exposure to ethanol. *Gastroenterology.* 1995;108(1):218-24.

[45] Bode, C., Bode, J. C. Activation of the innate immune system and alcoholic liver disease: effects of ethanol per se or enhanced intestinal translocation of bacterial toxins induced by ethanol? *Alcohol. Clin. Exp. Res.* 2005;29(11 Suppl.):166S-71S.

[46] Hritz, I., Mandrekar, P., Velayudham, A., Catalano, D., Dolganiuc, A., Kodys, K., Kurt-Jones, E., Szabo, G. The critical role of toll-like receptor (TLR) 4 in alcoholic liver disease is independent of the common TLR adapter MyD88. *Hepatology.* 2008;48(4):1224-31.

[47] Bala, S., Marcos, M., Gattu, A., Catalano, D., Szabo, G. Acute binge drinking increases serum endotoxin and bacterial DNA levels in healthy individuals. *PLoS One.* 2014;9(5):e96864.

[48] Inokuchi, S., Tsukamoto, H., Park, E., Liu, Z. X., Brenner, D. A., Seki, E. Toll-like receptor 4 mediates alcohol-induced steatohepatitis through bone marrow-derived and endogenous liver cells in mice. *Alcohol. Clin. Exp. Res.* 2011;35(8):1509-18.

[49] Garcia-Martinez, I., Shaker, M. E., Mehal, W. Z. Therapeutic Opportunities in Damage-Associated Molecular Pattern-Driven

Metabolic Diseases. *Antioxid. Redox Signal.* 2015 [Epub. ahead of print].

[50] Ouyang, X., Ghani, A., Malik, A., Wilder, T., Colegio, O. R., Flavell, R. A., Cronstein, B. N., Mehal, W. Z. Adenosine is required for sustained inflammasome activation via the A_2A receptor and the HIF-1α pathway. *Nat. Commun.* 2013;4:2909.

[51] Lamkanfi, M., Kanneganti, T. D., Franchi, L., Núñez, G. Caspase-1 inflammasomes in infection and inflammation. *J. Leukoc. Biol.* 2007;82 (2):220-5.

[52] Kanneganti, T. D., Ozören, N., Body-Malapel, M., Amer, A., Park, J. H., Franchi, L., Whitfield, J., Barchet, W., Colonna, M., Vandenabeele, P., Bertin, J., Coyle, A., Grant, E. P., Akira, S., Núñez, G. Bacterial RNA and small antiviral compounds activate caspase-1 through cryopyrin/ Nalp3. *Nature.* 2006;440(7081):233-6.

[53] Mariathasan, S., Weiss, D. S., Newton, K., McBride, J., O'Rourke, K., Roose-Girma, M., Lee, W. P., Weinrauch, Y., Monack, D. M., Dixit, V. M. Cryopyrin activates the inflammasome in response to toxins and ATP. *Nature.* 2006;440(7081):228-32.

[54] Zamboni, D. S., Kobayashi, K. S., Kohlsdorf, T., Ogura, Y., Long, E. M., Vance, R. E., Kuida, K., Mariathasan, S., Dixit, V. M., Flavell, R. A., Dietrich, W. F., Roy, C. R. The Birc1e cytosolic pattern-recognition receptor contributes to the detection and control of Legionella pneumophila infection. *Nat. Immunol.* 2006;7(3):318-25.

[55] Amer, A., Franchi, L., Kanneganti, T. D., Body-Malapel, M., Ozören, N., Brady, G., Meshinchi, S., Jagirdar, R., Gewirtz, A., Akira, S., Núñez, G. Regulation of Legionella phagosome maturation and infection through flagellin and host Ipaf. *J. Biol. Chem.* 2006;281(46):35217-23.

[56] Miao, E. A., Alpuche-Aranda, C. M., Dors, M., Clark, A. E., Bader, M. W., Miller, S. I., Aderem, A. Cytoplasmic flagellin activates caspase-1 and secretion of interleukin 1beta via Ipaf. *Nat. Immunol.* 2006;7(6):569-75.

[57] Miao, E. A., Ernst, R. K., Dors, M., Mao, D. P., Aderem, A. Pseudomonas aeruginosa activates caspase 1 through Ipaf. *Proc. Natl. Acad. Sci. US.* 2008;105(7):2562-7.

[58] Franchi, L., Stoolman, J., Kanneganti, T. D., Verma, A., Ramphal, R., Núñez, G. Critical role for Ipaf in Pseudomonas aeruginosa-induced caspase-1 activation. *Eur. J. Immunol.* 2007;37(11):3030-9.

[59] Franchi, L., Warner, N., Viani, K., Nuñez, G. Function of Nod-like receptors in microbial recognition and host defense. *Immunol. Rev.* 2009;227(1):106-28.

[60] DeSantis, D. A., Ko, C. W., Liu, Y., Liu, X., Hise, A. G., Nunez, G., Croniger, C. M. Alcohol-induced liver injury is modulated by Nlrp3 and Nlrc4 inflammasomes in mice. *Mediators Inflamm.* 2013; 2013:751374.

[61] Friedman, S. L. Stellate cells: a moving target in hepatic fibrogenesis. *Hepatology.* 2004;40:1041-1043.

[62] Watanabe, A., Sohail, M. A., Gomes, D. A., Hashmi, A., Nagata, J., Sutterwala, F. S., Mahmood, S., Jhandier, M. N., Shi, Y., Flavell, R. A., Mehal, W. Z. Inflammasome-mediated regulation of hepatic stellate cells. *Am. J. Physiol. Gastrointest. Liver Physiol.* 2009; 296(6):G1248-57.

[63] Chan, E. S., Montesinos, M. C., Fernandez, P., Desai, A., Delano, D. L., Yee, H., Reiss, A. B., Pillinger, M. H., Chen, J. F., Schwarzschild, M. A., Friedman, S. L., Cronstein, B. N. Adenosine A(2A) receptors play a role in the pathogenesis of hepatic cirrhosis. *Br. J. Pharmacol.* 2006;148 (8):1144-55.

[64] Peng, Z., Borea, P. A., Varani, K., Wilder, T., Yee, H., Chiriboga, L., Blackburn, M. R., Azzena, G., Resta, G., Cronstein, B. N. Adenosine signaling contributes to ethanol-induced fatty liver in mice. *J. Clin. Invest.* 2009;119(3):582-94.

[65] Kim, Y. O., Stoll, M., Hebich, B., Robson, S., Schuppan, D. Adenosine 2B receptor antagonism alleviates liver fibrosis progression and induces mild fibrosis regression. *Z. Gastroenterol.* 2012; 50-K031.

[66] Latasa, M. U., Gil-Puig, C., Fernández-Barrena, M. G., Rodríguez-Ortigosa, C. M., Banales, J. M., Urtasun, R., Goñi, S., Méndez, M., Arcelus, S., Juanarena, N., Recio, J. A., Lotersztajn, S., Prieto, J., Berasain, C., Corrales, F. J., Lecanda, J., Avila, M. A. Oral methylthioadenosine administration attenuates fibrosis and chronic liver disease progression in Mdr2-/- mice. *PLoS One.* 2010;5(12):e15690.

[67] Peng, Z., Fernandez, P., Wilder, T., Yee, H., Chiriboga, L., Chan, E. S., Cronstein, B. N. Ecto-5'-nucleotidase (CD73)-mediated extracellular adenosine production plays a critical role in hepatic fibrosis. *FASEB J.* 2008;22:2263-2272.

[68] Andrade, C. M., Lopez, P. L., Noronha, B. T., Wink, M. R., Borojevic, R., Margis, R., Lenz, G., Battastini, A. M., Guma, F. C. Ecto-5'-nucleotidase/CD73 knockdown increases cell migration and mRNA

level of collagen I in a hepatic stellate cell line. *Cell Tissue Res*. 2011 May;344(2):279-86.

[69] Feld, J. J., Lavoie, É. G., Michel, F., Dranoff, J. A. I drink for my liver, Doc: emerging evidence that coffee prevents cirrhosis. *F1000Res*. 2015; 4:95.

In: Alcohol and the Liver
Editor: Gerond Lake-Bakaar
ISBN: 978-1-63484-400-0

Chapter 4

ASSESSMENT OF MALNUTRITION IN ALCOHOLIC LIVER DISEASE

Audrey Paradis**, *MS, RD, LDN, CNSC
Transplant Dietitian at Beth Israel Deaconess Medical Center,
Boston, MA, US

ABSTRACT

Defining malnutrition in individuals with liver disease is a challenge. Many tools that are typically used to assess nutrition status are not reliable indicators and should be used with caution. This chapter explores the current methods of assessing nutrition status and offers insight into the appropriate assessment of malnutrition in patients with alcoholic liver disease.

INTRODUCTION

The majority of individuals with alcoholic liver disease (ALD) exhibit one or more signs of malnutrition [1]. Malnutrition has found to be more prevalent in ALD compared to those with non-alcoholic liver disease [2, 3, 4]. Protein energy malnutrition (PEM) in this population often increases risk factors for

* Email: aparadis@BIDMC.harvard.edu.

such complications as hepatic encephalopathy, infections, ascites and variceal bleeding [1].

Factors contributing to the decline in nutrition status in alcoholic liver disease include altered taste change, depressed appetite, early satiety, malabsorption of nutrients, decreased hepatic protein synthesis, alteration in metabolism and inadequate energy and protein consumption.

Challenges in Assessing Nutrition Status

It is common that cirrhotics demonstrate a degree of physical evidence on visual exam including muscle and subcutaneous fat wasting. Evaluating for malnutrition is often difficult due to the skewing of a multitude of objective parameters resulting from the effects of chronic alcohol use with concurrent liver disease. Nutrition status is heavily dependent on the duration of alcohol abuse and degree of underlying liver disease along with notably poor intake for weeks to even years. Malnutrition is often underdiagnosed, especially in the early stages of liver disease when physical losses are masked by fluid retention [5]. In cirrhotics with Child-Pugh stage A, the prevalence of PEM increases to 20%, while those with stage C can further increase to 60% and can even reach to 100% in those with alcoholic hepatitis [6, 7].

Methods of Assessing Nutrition Status

It is important that the proper steps are taken to ensure that all alcoholic liver disease patients are assessed to provide the appropriate medical and nutrition therapy. There is currently no gold standard for diagnosing malnutrition in ALD, but interpreting a combination of objective and subjective data should be included when assessing nutrition status. A comprehensive assessment of nutrition status in ALD should include physical assessment, dietary history, anthropometric measures and laboratory values. Other more sophisticated tests are available, but often are not realistic in the inpatient or outpatient settings and are rather costly, time consuming and limited to research.

The Academy of Nutrition and Dietetics (AND) and the American Society of Parenteral and Enteral Nutrition (A.S.P.E.N.) have collaborated to help standardize the diagnosis of malnutrition. According to their Consensus

Statement on Malnutrition, six characteristics have been named as criteria for malnutrition and include, insufficient energy intake, weight loss, loss of muscle mass, loss of subcutaneous fat, localized or generalized fluid accumulation and diminished functional status [8]. Meeting two or more of these criteria in a hospitalized patient would be considered evidence of malnutrition. The degree to which these patients meet the criteria allows for classifications of moderate to severe malnutrition.

NUTRITION INTAKE

Assessment of energy and protein intake is an important source of information as to an individual's recent and long term dietary history. This can be accomplished both in the inpatient and outpatient settings by a skilled registered dietitian using dietary recall. Asking about average diet, food habits, meal and snack pattern, restaurant eating, food frequency and beverage in take should be thoroughly assessed. Although subjective and limited by mental capacity in some, it can provide a quick snapshot of nutrient intake and reveal under or over consumption of macronutrients and potential deficiencies. Family members can also pose as a great tool in providing more insight when patients are encephalopathic.

SUBJECTIVE GLOBAL ASSESSMENT

Another more comprehensive approach to assessing nutrition status is to use Subjective Global Assessment (SGA). This method involves detailed weight and dietary history, current gastrointestinal symptoms and physical activity as an evaluation tool. This then allows a rating of individuals as either "well-nourished," "moderately malnourished," or "severely malnourished." According to multiple studies, SGA lacks sensitivity when evaluating those with alcoholic liver disease and underestimated prevalence of malnutrition, especially when in an earlier stage of liver disease [9, 10, 11, 12]. One study did however show that worsening of SGA status appeared to increase in the late stages of cirrhosis and especially in the alcoholic group [4]. Based on these findings, this suggests SGA would not be a helpful tool in assessing for malnutrition in the early stages of alcoholic liver disease.

Weight

Weight is not a reliable indicator of malnutrition as fluid retention is typically present due to ascites an/or edema. Frequent paracenteses can cause significant fluctuations in weight with some individuals requiring therapeutic taps several times per week. Noting post-paracentesis weight can be helpful in monitoring trends if similar amounts of fluid is removed. Body Mass Index (BMI) when calculated using height and weight in the presence of ascites and/or edema may produce a falsely elevated value and therefore, is also unreliable in assessing for malnutrition. Exceptions include in instances when edema and/or ascites is absent or when close estimations of fluid can be subtracted to provide correction [10, 13].

Biochemical Markers

Using biochemical markers such as acute phase proteins, serum albumin or prealbumin levels to assess visceral protein status is unreliable in the presence of ascites/edema as it is highly affected by fluid status. Prijatmoko et al. [14], noted that the correlation between serum albumin and nitrogen index was weak because the changes in serum albumin levels may largely reflect fluctuations in total body water. Decreased protein synthesis by the liver causing hypoalbuminemia is an expected outcome in the setting of ALD. Decreasing levels of albumin and prealbumin have been found to correlate with different stages of cirrhosis with no significant difference between non-alcoholic and alcoholic groups as observed in a Thailand Study [4]. Inflammation has been identified to be an underlying risk for malnutrition and negatively affects acute phase protein levels by causing a falsely low level. Currently, the Academy of Nutrition and Dietetics and the American Society for Enteral and Parenteral Nutrition (A.S.P.E.N.) do not propose any specific inflammatory markers for diagnosis [8].

24-Hour Creatinine Excretion

Measurements of 24-hour creatinine excretion is an indirect way of estimating body muscle mass. Andersen et al. [15], found a close correlation between muscle strength of the ankle, knee, hip, shoulder, elbow and wrist and the lean body mass estimated by creatinine excretion with the severity of weakness closely related to malnutrition. Two other studies found that lean body mass may be falsely low in cirrhotic individuals as creatinine is synthesized by the liver [16] and in those with renal dysfunction caused by extrarenal excretion and recycling of creatinine to creatine, respectively [17]. However, Neilsen et al. [18], found that three 24-hour creatinine excretion measurements were reliable indicators of lean body mass in the presence of normal renal function. This suggests that using 24-hour creatinine excretion could be a helpful predictor of nutrition status in early stages of liver disease. Retrospective studies noted that hepatorenal syndrome (HRS) is seen in approximately 17% of cirrhotic patients with ascites while it is present in >50% of end-stage liver disease patients [19].

Physical Assessment

Physical exam is very appropriate in this population. While there can be overt signs of under-nutrition immediately upon exam, it is important to get a broad observation to monitor trends and provide clues of other potential nutritional deficiencies. Muscle wasting/atrophy can be seen as the loss of bulk and tone. It can be a result of numerous factors including acute or chronic inflammatory illness, aging, decreased physical activity, starvation and neurological impairment [20]. Observing the upper body is more useful for evaluating and identifying fat and muscle losses as it often less affected by edema and considered to be a good reflection of overall muscle mass [21]. Palpating for muscle losses in the temporal, clavicular and scapular region and for fat loss in the orbital region of the upper body can help identify and grade the severity of malnutrition which is exceptionally useful in these patients stricken with edema and ascites.

Hand Grip Strength

Loss of muscle inevitably results in decreased weight and increased weakness and can be reflected in strength testing. Hand grip strength (HGS) as recorded by dynamometry, is a validated method and is feasible in the inpatient and outpatient setting. When coupled with arm circumference, it has been shown to have sensitivity of 94% and negative predictive value of 97% in identifying depleted body cell mass in cirrhotics [10]. It is also considered the best modality for predicting major complications at 1 year in undernourished cirrhotic patients [11] and has been found to be an independent predictor of poor outcomes and mortality of hospitalized patients [22]. In a study comparing the use of HGS and SGA to assess nutritional status in cirrhotic patients, HGS was considered superior with the prevalence of malnutrition found to be 28% by SGA and 63% by HGS [11]. HGS should be considered for the assessment of nutrition status in mild cirrhosis as changes in strength have been seen in early liver disease, whereas, SGA could be more appropriately used in late stages of liver disease [2].

Tricep Skinfold Test

Tricep Skinfold (TSF) is an anthropometric measure that estimates body fat and is considered the most predictive of all body sites to assess fat stores [24]. TSF provides an indication of energy reserves available in the form of fat stores. The use is based on the assumption that the thickness of the subcutaneous adipose tissue is proportional to total body fat. It is important to note that the presence of generalized edema may prevent accurate estimation of fat free mass [25]. According to a study performed by Simpson et al. it was not recommended to use TSF when in the presence of edema [26]. Interestingly, in another study, it was found that fat mass when measured by tricep skinfold test was significantly lower in an alcoholic group as compared to the non-alcoholic group suggesting that fat wasting can be seen in this population [4]. Tricep skin fold thickness and mid-arm circumference decrease significantly according to the Child score, a positive correlation was found between these two parameters and the severity of cirrhosis [27].

Mid-Arm Circumference

Mid-arm circumference (MAC) is an anthropometric measurement that reflects the reserves of muscle protein [24]. Mid upper arm muscle circumference (MAMC) assesses lean body mass, but may be another measure affected by edema decreasing its reliability [25]. It is derived from MAC and TSF in the equation that follows: MAMC = MAC – (3.14 x TSF). Nielson et al. found that in patients with ascites or edema, or both, the correlation between lean body mass and MAMC was poor [18]. Also, it should be noted that several studies have shown that 20-30% of healthy controls were consider malnourished when using MAMC [28].

Advanced Composition Tests

Duel-energy x-ray absorptiometry (DEXA) and bioelectrical impedance analysis (BIA) are advanced tests that assess body composition. They are both costly and often limited to research, but advantageously, BIA can be performed at the bedside and holds less of a costly burden. These methods measure fat free mass by estimating both body water and body protein compartments and may fail to show a significant reduction in body protein given increased total body water (TBW) as seen in cirrhotics with ascites and edema. In a study from 2006, it was found that DEXA perceived the increased extracellular water (ECW) as a change in lean body mass, which masked the decrease in body cell mass seen in liver patients. The authors of this study suggest that with combining DEXA and body water measurements, it may be possible to measure fat, mineral and water compartments independently, thereby deriving an estimate of body cell mass independent of hydration and increasing accuracy of body composition analysis [12]. BIA is a non-invasive way of measuring lean body and fat stores based on the principle that conduction through fat tissue tends to be decreased due to increased resistance, whereas, a more rapid conduction will be seen through water. According to the European Society of Parenteral and Enteral Nutrition (ESPEN), BIA is a reliable bedside tool to evaluate body composition, but is limited in liver patients with abnormal fluid distribution [29]. Pirlich et al. found that BIA provides reliable estimates of body cell mass in groups of patients with large amounts of ascites and is superior to other bedside techniques, such as anthropometry or urinary creatinine excretion [30]. Schloerb et al. [31], reports little success when using BIA to determine total body water (TBW) in patients with liver disease and anasarca in efforts to estimate body cell mass to serve as a reference for "dry weight" to help monitor for true weight changes. One recent study concludes that BIA presents with poor accuracy and high variability, but interestingly was found to be the only method that was statistically significant when compared to Child-Pugh score [32]. Lehnert et al. [33], suggests that this tool could be useful in monitoring and following the nutritional state of a patient as their progression of liver disease evolves. Future studies using BIA should be considered moving forward given its low margin of error [32]. Body composition changes in alcoholic cirrhosis patients requires the use of direct methods such as in vivo neutron activation analysis and DEXA according to Prijatmoko et al. [14].

In vivo neutron activation analysis (IVNAA) provides more of a sensitive measure of total body protein and is thought to be useful when assessing for malnutrition in the early stages of alcoholic cirrhosis [14]. This information could be helpful in providing early nutrition interventions and supplementation for those who otherwise would have been overlooked as potentially at risk for malnutrition. Unfortunately, this type of analysis is limited to research and few centers exist in the United States.

Conclusion

Assessing nutrition status in ALD requires a multitude of approaches. No one method alone can diagnose malnutrition. Multiple recommendations exist. ESPEN [8] suggests using bedside methods such as SGA and/or anthropometry parameters to identify patients at nutritional risk and BIA to quantify under-nutrition despite the limitations with ascites. Others suggest using three 24-hour creatinine excretions in conjunction with dietary recalls for most accurate diagnosing [18].

In any case, it can be suggested that Child Pugh A and B patients would likely benefit from complex nutritional assessment as they often show no obvious signs of malnutrition and are often undiagnosed [5], but could gain from early intervention. In the later stages of liver disease such as in Child Pugh C class, these patients are visibly malnourished and it would be imperative to initiate nutritional intervention as soon as possible.

References

[1] Mendenhall CL, Roselle GA, Gartide P, Moritz T. Relationship of protein calorie malnutrition to alcoholic liver disease: a reexamination of data from two Veterans Administration Cooperative Studies. *Alc. Clin. Res.* 1995; 19(3):635-41.

[2] Marsano L, McClain CJ. Nutrition and alcoholic liver disease. *J. Parenter Enteral Nutr.* 1991;15(3):337-44.

[3] Peng S, Plank LD, McCall JL, Gillanders LK, McIlroy K, Gane EJ. Cabre E, Gassull MA. Body composition, muscle function, and energy

expenditure in patients with liver cirrhosis: a comprehensive study. *Am. J. Clin. Nutr.* 2007;859(5):1257-66.

[4] Roongpisuthipong C, Sobhonslidsuk A, Nantiruj K, Songchitsomboon S. Nutrition Assessment in Various Stages of Liver Cirrhosis. *Nutrition* 2001;17(9):761-765.

[5] Cabre E, Gassull MA. Nutrition in chronic liver disease and liver transplantation. *Curr. Opin. Clin. Nutr. Metab. Care* 1998;1(5):423-30.

[6] Muller MJ, Lautz HU, Plogmann B, Burger M, Korber J, Schmidt FW. Energy expenditure and substrate oxidation in patients with cirrhosis: the impact of cause, clinical staging and nutritional state. *Hepatology* 1992;15(5):782-94.

[7] Mendenahall CL, Anderson S, Weesner RE, Goldberg SL, Crolic KA. Protein-calorie malnutrition associated with alcoholic hepatitis. Veterans Administration Cooperative Study Group on Alcoholic Hepatitis. *Am. J. Med.* 1984; 76(2):211-22.

[8] White JV, Guenter P, Jensen G, Malone A, Schofield M, the Academy Malnutrition Work Group, the A.S.P.E.N. Malnutrition Task Force, the A.S.P.E.N. Board of Directors. Consensus Statement of the Academy of Nutrition and Dietetics/American Society for Pareneteral and Enteral Nutrition: Characteristics Recommended for the Identification and Documentation of Adult Malnutrition. *J. Acad. Nutr. Diet.* 2012;36(3):275-283.

[9] Naveau S, Belda E, Borotto E, Genuist F, Chaput JC. Comparison of clinical judgment and anthropometric parameters for evaluating nutritional status in patients with alcoholic liver disease. *J. Hepatol.* 1995; 23(2): 234–235.

[10] Figueiredo FA, Dickson ER, Pasha TM, Porayko MK, Therneau TM, Malinchoc M, DiCecco SR, Francisco-Ziller NM, Kasparova P, Charlton MR.

[11] Utility of standard nutrition parameters in detecting body cell mass depletion in patients with end-stage liver disease. *Liver Transpl.* 2000;6(5):575-81.

[12] Alvarez-da-silva MR, Reverbel da Silveira T. Comparison between handgrip strength subjective global assessment and prognostic nutritional index in assessing malnutrition and predicting clinical outcome in cirrhotic outpatients. *Nutrition* 2005;21(2):113-17.

[13] Figueiredo FA, Perez RM, Freitas MM, Kondo M. Comparison of three methods of nutritional assessment in liver cirrhosis: subjective global

In: Alcohol and the Liver
Editor: Gerond Lake-Bakaar
ISBN: 978-1-63484-400-0

Chapter 5

VITAMINS AND SUPPLEMENTS IN ALCOHOLIC LIVER DISEASE

Katelyn R. Richards*[*], *PharmD
Clinical Pharmacist – Solid Organ Transplant,
Beth Israel Deaconess Medical Center, Boston, MA, US

ABSTRACT

Significant malnutrition in alcoholics is caused by reduced dietary intake as well as alternations in absorption of essential vitamins and nutrients. Malabsorption may be due to alcohol's direct effect on the small intestine inhibiting the absorption of amino acids, lipids and vitamins. A decrease in biliary output can also play a role in the malabsorption of fat soluble vitamins. However, if dietary intake is reconciled, the alternations in absorption normalize.

INTRODUCTION

Malnutrition in alcoholics is caused by reduced dietary intake as well as alterations in absorption of essential vitamins and nutrients [10, 8, 45, 31, 19]. Malabsorption may be due to alcohol's direct effect on the small intestine inhibiting the absorption of amino acids, lipids and vitamins. A decrease in

[*] Email: krrichar@bidmc.harvard.edu.

biliary output can also play a role in the malabsorption of fat soluble vitamins [19, 8]. However, if dietary intake is reconciled, the alternations in absorption normalize [10, 19].

Water Soluble Vitamins

Vitamin B_1 (Thiamine)

Thiamine deficiency is one of the most common vitamin deficiencies in alcoholics and can occur after 2-3 weeks of inadequate dietary intake [32]. The deficiency is due to both decreased intake as well as malabsorption of the vitamin in the small intestine [8, 10]. Alcohol has been shown to inhibit two transporters in the small intestine used by thiamine, thiamine transporters 1 and 2, and also decrease the formation of active thiamine, thiamine diphosphate [41]. Thiamine deficiency can lead to serious neurologic diseases including Wernicke-Korsakoff syndrome and Beri-Beri disease [45].

In the United States, the recommended daily allowance (RDA) of thiamine in adults is 1.2 mg daily for males and 1.1 mg daily for females [23]. In healthy individuals, thiamine is poorly absorbed with only about 4.5 mg absorbed following a single oral dose of 30 mg [47, 48]. In the setting of alcoholism, absorption of thiamine can be even more variable. In adults with alcohol-induced malnutrition, a single dose of oral thiamine yields only 0.8 mg or less absorption after acute alcohol consumption [12]. Thus, parenteral administration is preferred for subjects who need rapid repletion of thiamine. In the presence of established Wernicke's encephalopathy, 500 mg of intravenous or intramuscular thiamine for 3-5 days may be administered [48, 12]. However this recommendation is based on uncontrolled studies and the appropriate dose of thiamine to prevent and treat Werinicke-Korsakoff Syndrome has yet to be established [13, 48]. In an effort to prevent Wernicke's encephalopathy, most clinicians start patients with alcoholic liver disease on maintenance thiamine 100 mg orally daily [16, 37].

Vitamin B_2 (Riboflavin)

Riboflavin deficiency can be observed in alcoholism and may be directly related to the degree of liver injury. The influence of alcohol on ribavirin absorption in the small intestine is unknown. Subjects with cirrhosis have a higher frequency of riboflavin deficiency [29]. The assessment of riboflavin deficiency can be difficult due to the influence of short-term dietary intake on the concentration in blood and urine. Flavin adenine dinucleotide (FAD), one of the coenzymes of riboflavin, activates glutathione reductase. Glutathione reductase can be measured to assess riboflavin deficiency [49]. In a study by Rosenthal and colleagues, 11 of 22 subjects with severe alcoholism admitted to the hospital were shown to have riboflavin deficiency by measuring the activity of glutathione reductase. However, none of the riboflavin-deficient subjects exhibited symptoms of riboflavin deficiency. Riboflavin 5 mg, administered intramuscularly daily for 2-7 days corrected the laboratory evidence of riboflavin deficiency [42]. Given the lack of symptoms, it is possible the number of alcoholic subjects with riboflavin deficiency is higher than reported. However, the clinical significance of riboflavin deficiency in alcoholism has yet to be defined.

Vitamin B_3 (Niacin)

Niacin deficiency in alcohol abusers is due to reduced nutritional intake as well as impaired absorption. Alcohol may also decrease the formation of niacin precursors by inhibiting the liver enzyme tryptophan 2,3-dioxygenase [3]. Niacin deficiency can lead to alcoholic pellagra, a significantly less common disease than Wernicke-Korsakoff Syndrome. It has been suggested that a routine multivitamin administration is associated with a reduced incidence of this disease [12].

Niacin and nicotinamide (another version of niacin) play a critical role in the degradation of alcohol by the liver. Niacin is the precursor to the cofactor nicotinamide adenine dinucleotide (NAD+). Alcohol dehydrogenase uses NAD+ to metabolize alcohol to acetaldehyde and at the same time converts NAD+ to its reduced from NADH [20, 27, 38]. The result of this process decreases NAD+ thus affecting other reactions including fatty acid oxidation which contributes to the development of alcoholic liver disease [27]. In an animal study, the administration of niacin successfully restored NAD+ levels in the liver and reduced alcohol-induced hepatic steatosis [30]. However, niacin supplementation has been shown to cause mild to moderate elevations in serum aminotransferase. Significant hepatotoxicity is rare with niacin but can be common when high doses (>3 g per day) and the sustained release form are utilized [15]. Niacin undergoes methylation within and outside the liver. Excessive niacin can lead to methylation abnormalities which may also lead to liver toxicity [27]. Further studies are needed to define the most safe and effective dose of niacin to reduce alcohol-induced hepatic steatosis.

Vitamin B_6 (Pyridoxine)

Approximately 50% of alcoholics are deficient in pyridoxine and pyridoxal-5'-phosphate (PLP), the active coenzyme of pyridoxine [12, 45]. Pyridoxine is absorbed primarily in the small intestine and is transferred to the liver where PLP is primarily synthesized [50]. Pyridoxine deficiency in alcohol abusers may be due to reduced dietary intake and the inhibitory effect of alcohol on PLP [8, 45, 50]. Interestingly, as long as alcohol continues to be consumed PLP levels remain low despite parenteral supplementation. In animal studies, it was discovered that acetaldehyde may accelerate PLP metabolism in the liver [50]. Additionally, alcohol may also displace protein-bound PLP which is then phosphorylated to an inactive form [45].

It has been suggested that pyridoxine deficiency may be linked to alcohol-withdrawal seizures and peripheral neuropathy. Pyridoxine is the coenzyme for glutamic acid decarboxylase (GAD) which is the enzyme involved in creating gamma aminobutyric acid (GABA), an inhibitory neurotransmitter [12]. The causative relationship between pyridoxine deficiency and alcohol-induced seizures is yet to be defined in the literature.

Pyridoxine deficiency may also contribute to the progression of alcoholic liver disease. Pyridoxine is an important cofactor for the metabolism of homocysteine to glutathione and, as a result, a regulator of methionine metabolism. The lack of pyridoxine-dependent enzyme activity may lead to worsening fibrosis and alcoholic liver disease [33, 34].

The RDA of pyridoxine for adults (19-50 years old) is 1.3 mg for males and 1.2 mg for females [23]. Vitamin B complex daily supplementation in alcohol abusers is a reasonable recommendation but continued alcohol use may impede the benefits of pyridoxine supplementation.

Vitamin B_9 (Folic Acid/Folate)

Up to 80% of alcoholics have been found to be deficient in folate [33, 21, 22]. However, after folate fortification of grains in 1998 in the United States, the frequency of significant folate deficiency decreased. Chronic alcoholics continue to have a lower folate level when compared to healthy controls but significant folate deficiency is rare [33].

Low serum folate is caused by inadequate dietary intake and reduced jejunal uptake [21, 22]. Homeostasis of folate in the body may also be interrupted by alcohol exposure. In animal studies, chronic alcohol reduced the activity of glutamate carboxypeptidase (GCPII) and reduced folate carrier (RFC) which are needed for successful transfer of folate across the brush border in the intestine. Acute alcohol intake does not appear to have a significant effect on absorption of folate in the small intestine but may decrease serum folate levels for a short period of time. The mechanism to explain this phenomenon is yet to be defined [33]. In contrast, chronic alcohol abuse can reduce liver uptake and increase renal excretion of folate [21, 22].

Folate is essential for methionine synthesis in the liver. Among other activities, methionine regulates homocysteine levels in the liver, possesses antioxidant properties, and aids in the formation of DNA. Methionine is then converted to S-adenosylmethionine (SAM) which is a methyl donor for reactions involving DNA, proteins and hormones. Inadequate methionine decreases the synthesis of SAM which has been linked to the development of alcoholic liver disease [21, 22]. In animal studies, the onset of alcoholic liver disease was accelerated in pigs being fed a folate deficient diet when compared to pigs fed a folate sufficient diet [21]. This data suggests dietary intake of folate may impact the speed at which alcoholic liver disease develops [21, 33]. Interestingly, the impact of methionine deficiency leading to decreased methylation of DNA in the liver may increase the risk of hepatocellular carcinoma [33].

The effect of folate supplementation on alcoholic liver disease has been investigated in animal studies and has shown decreased homocysteine levels [33]. Human studies, however, are lacking. Given the potential impact of folate supplementation on the development of alcoholic liver disease, most clinicians recommend folic acid 1 mg daily for chronic alcohol abusers [37, 16].

Vitamin B_{12} (Cobalamin)

Cobalamin is transported from the peripheral tissues by transcobalamin II (TC II) and transcobalamin I (TC I) to the liver where it's primarily stored [17, 25]. In alcoholic liver disease, cobalamin leaks from the liver into plasma [4]. Serum cobalamin levels in alcoholics tend to be higher when compared to healthy controls and, in response the total cobalamin concentration in liver tissue is decreased [4, 5]. In fact, elevations in serum cobalamin levels can predict the degree of liver injury and risk of mortality [4].

Cobalamin is a cofactor for methionine synthesis in the liver [22]. In severe alcoholic liver disease, methionine synthesis is decreased leading to decreased production of SAM. Insufficient concentration of SAM in the liver may worsen the degree of alcoholic liver disease [33, 4].

The impact of vitamin B_{12} supplementation is unclear. Administering high intramuscular doses of vitamin B_{12} has been hypothesized to temporarily decrease the need for cobalamin transporters and increase stores in the liver. Once cobalamin stores are adequate in the liver, synthesis of DNA may normalize and augment liver regeneration [4].

Vitamin C (Ascorbic Acid)

Alcoholic liver disease has been associated with ascorbic acid deficiency [6]. Additionally, alcoholics without evidence of liver disease may also experience ascorbic acid deficiency [28]. This deficiency is due to inadequate dietary intake, increased urinary excretion, and insufficient absorption [8].

Although rare, ascorbic acid deficiency in alcoholics can lead to scurvy [43]. Recommendation for supplementation of ascorbic acid is not clear in the literature. The RDA recommendation for adults ranges between 75 and 90 mg which is typically available in a regular multivitamin [24].

Ascorbic acid supplementation may play a role in reducing oxidative stress in alcoholic liver disease [1, 2].

Fat Soluble Vitamins

Vitamin A (Retinol)

Fat soluble vitamins are typically decreased in severe alcoholic liver disease due to impaired intestinal absorption from pancreatic insufficiency and cholestasis [8]. Deficiency in vitamin A can be seen in 50% of patients with alcoholic cirrhosis [7]. Vitamin A deficiency in alcoholic liver disease is from inadequate dietary intake, impaired absorption and decreased liver stores [16]. Alcohol can enhance the activity of enzymes in the liver to breakdown retinol, promote secretion of vitamin A from the liver, and, in severe alcoholic liver disease, impair the conversion of beta-carotene to retinol [31]. Similar to alcohol metabolism, retinol undergoes oxidation to form retinaldehyde then retinoic acid. The competition for enzymatic metabolism results in reduced vitamin A activity [19, 11]. Interestingly, serum levels of beta-carotene remains normal in the setting of vitamin A deficiency suggesting the liver is unable to take up beta-carotene and/or convert it to retinol effectively when the liver is diseased [31].

Vitamin A deficiency can lead to night blindness, impaired immune function, and increased risk of hepatic fibrosis [16]. Vitamin A is primarily stored in stellate cells in the liver and when these cells are activated, vitamin A stores are decreased and can lead to production of collagen and fibrosis [7]. The alterations of vitamin A and beta-carotene by alcohol may contribute to the development of worsening liver disease [31]. Supplementing vitamin A deficiency is not recommended due to the difficulty in assessing true vitamin A deficiency (vitamin A plasma concentration is not reflective of tissue concentration), high doses of vitamin A can be hepatotoxic, and the continued use of alcohol can promote the toxic effects of vitamin A supplements [31]. Alcohol induces cytochrome P450 2E1 isoenzyme which in the presence of vitamin A can lead to hepatotoxic metabolites [45]. In patients with severe vitamin A deficiency resulting in night blindness, a small dose of vitamin A (2 mg per day) may be considered with extreme caution and only in subjects who abstain from alcohol use [31, 16].

Vitamin E (Tocopherol)

In alcoholic subjects, vitamin E levels diminish as the severity of liver injury worsens [14]. Consistent with all fat soluble vitamins, vitamin E absorption can be significantly decreased in the setting of pancreatic insufficiency and alcoholic liver disease [16].

In alcoholic liver disease, there is an increase in free radicals causing oxidative stress in the liver. Vitamin E is an antioxidant that can prevent lipid peroxidation and scavenge free radicals [19]. However, studies with vitamin E supplementation in liver disease do not reflect improvement in liver function. Long term vitamin E supplementation was evaluated in a randomized controlled double blinded study using subjects with decompensated alcoholic cirrhosis. Vitamin E 500 mg daily for 1 year did not influence mortality, hospitalization, or laboratory values even though the vitamin E serum level was significantly increased [14]. Similarly, vitamin E supplementation in mild to moderate alcoholic hepatitis did lead to improvement of liver function or mortality at 3 months when compared to placebo [35].

In addition to the lack of evidence for vitamin E supplementation, vitamin E can also increase the risk of bleeding and in a patient population with known coagulopathy, adding vitamin E may increase that risk [46].

Vitamin D

In addition to malabsorption in the setting of alcoholic liver disease and pancreatic insufficiency, serum vitamin D levels, 25-hydroxy-vitamin D, can also be affected by poor dietary intake and decreased sunlight exposure [16, 8]. To activate vitamin D it undergoes two steps the first being in the liver and the second being in the kidney. Vitamin D undergoes hydroxylation in the liver to form 25-hydroxyvitamin D which is then transferred to the kidney for the final activation step. In the setting of liver disease, vitamin D hydroxylation in the liver is diminished. As liver disease progresses, hydroxylation of vitamin D continues to lessen [16, 7]. Additionally, hepatic vitamin D binding protein, plasma carrier protein of 25-hydroxyvitamin D, production is decreased in end stage liver disease which may also contribute to vitamin D deficiency [7]. Significant vitamin D deficiency has been linked to poor outcomes for subjects with hepatitis C and increased mortality in subjects with chronic liver disease. It has been speculated that the impaired immune function in the absence of vitamin D may explain this observation [7]. Furthermore, the reduction in vitamin D activity may impact bone metabolism and lead to osteoporosis subjects with alcoholic liver disease [16].

Vitamin D supplementation may be considered for patients with an established deficiency. Options for supplementation include either cholecalciferol 400-800 IU per day or ergocalciferol 50,000 units per week. Vitamin D stores may be reassessed after 2-3 months of therapy [16].

Minerals and Trace Elements

Iron

Serum iron is often elevated in alcoholic liver disease due to increased absorption [10]. The non-carrier mediated paracellular route may be upregulated in chronic alcoholics which increases the absorption of iron [8]. In contrast, iron depletion can be seen in chronic alcoholics and may be secondary to blood loss related to complications of liver disease. Iron studies should be performed periodically to determine the quantity of iron needed, if any, in addition to the recommended multivitamin [16].

However, iron overload is a concern in alcoholic liver disease. Iron overload from increased intestinal absorption and transfusions coupled with continued alcohol consumption may promote fibrosis formation [16, 7]. Iron promotes an environment of oxidative stress through the production of free radicals and can lead to tissue injury in the liver [40]. In a large, national observational study, elevated transferrin-iron saturation was associated with the development of cirrhosis, especially with continued alcohol consumption [7].

Calcium and Magnesium

Absorption of calcium and magnesium may not be significantly affected by acute or chronic alcohol use [8]. In rat models calcium transport to the duodenum was reduced in the presence of alcohol [10] but human studies are lacking. The calcium deficiency observed in alcoholic liver disease may be due to inadequate dietary intake of calcium, vitamin D deficiency, and increased renal excretion [16, 18]. Low serum calcium may also be influenced by low magnesium and albumin in alcoholic liver disease [16]. Acute alcohol ingestion causes transient hypoparathyroidism leading to decreased parathyroid hormone (PTH) and increased urinary excretion of calcium and magnesium [44]. Increased urinary excretion of magnesium, diarrhea, and decreased dietary intake in chronic alcoholics can lead to hypomagnesemia [8, 10]. Newer literature suggests alcohol may impair transport and homeostasis of magnesium in the brain, skeletal muscle, heart and liver [7].

As with vitamin D deficiency, hypocalcemia from malnutrition can lead to osteoporosis [16, 44]. In subjects who are unable to increase dietary intake of calcium, calcium supplementation of 1000-1500 mg per day is recommended [16].

Magnesium deficiency can lead to insulin resistance which is observed in alcoholic liver disease as well as worsen hepatic damage caused by alcohol [7, 39]. The role of magnesium supplementation and its potential effects on liver enzyme activity in alcoholics was assessed in a randomized, parallel group, placebo-controlled, double-blinded trial. Subjects were randomized to receive either magnesium 500 mg daily or placebo for 8 weeks. The authors did not find a difference in activity of glutamyltransferase (S-GGT), aspartate-aminotransferase (AST) and alanine-aminotransferase (ALT) between the two groups. However, after controlling for baseline alcohol intake, age, body weight, change in alcohol intake, and baseline AST, AST levels were significantly lower in the group treated with magnesium [39]. This study demonstrates the potential effects of magnesium supplementation in compliant subjects but larger studies are required to further identify the role of magnesium in alcoholic liver disease.

Zinc

Zinc deficiency in chronic alcoholics is likely due to inadequate intake and increased renal excretion [16]. Studies are conflicting on the effect of alcohol abuse on absorption of zinc [8].

Zinc is required for cell development and differentiation as well as stimulation of osteoblastic bone formation [7, 18]. In addition, zinc is used to enhance vitamin A treatment in night blindness, augment hepatic encephalopathy treatment, and improve in immune function. Supplementation at a dose of 220 mg zinc sulfate in 1-3 divided doses may be considered for chronic alcoholics, especially those with complications such as night blindness and hepatic encephalopathy [16]. However, studies evaluating the effect of zinc on hepatic encephalopathy have only shown marginal improvement [9].

In addition, zinc may have a role in reducing alcoholic related liver injury. Recent animal studies have suggested zinc supplementation can prevent alcohol induced glutathione depletion and increase glutathione reductase activity. This increase in glutathione decreases the use of the alternative pathway for alcohol metabolism through CYP2E1 which will decrease the production of reactive oxidative stress thus reducing the liver injury incurred from alcohol [51, 26]. Zinc has also been linked to decreasing proinflammatory cytokine production in the liver and slowing hepatocyte death which may lead to a reduction in alcoholic-induced liver injury. The role of zinc supplementation in human subjects with liver disease from any cause has been explored in the literature. Studies illustrate an improvement of laboratory hepatic function tests, Child-Pugh score, and nutritional parameters following long-term zinc supplementation. However, further randomized studies are required to evaluate its effectiveness specifically in alcoholic liver disease [36].

References

[1] Abhilash PA, Hrikrishnan R, Indira M. Ascorbic acid supplementation down-regulates the alcohol induced oxidative stress, hepatic stellate cell activation, cytotoxicity and mRNA levels of selected fibrotic genes in guinea pigs. *Free Radic. Res.* 2012 Jan; 46(2):204-213.

[2] Abhilash PA, Harikrishnan R, Indira M. Ascorbic acid suppresses endotoxemia and NF-κB signaling cascade in alcoholic liver fibrosis in guinea pigs: a mechanistic approach. *Toxicol. Appl. Pharmacol.* 2014 Jan; 274:215-224.

[3] Badawy AAB. Pellagra and alcoholism: a biochemical perspective. *Alcohol Alcohol.* 2014 May; 49(3):238-250.

[4] Baker H, Frank O, DeAngelis B. Plasma vitamin B12 titres as indicators of disease severity and mortality of patients with alcoholic hepatitis. *Alcohol Alcohol.* 1987 Jan; 22:1-5.

[5] Baker H, Leevy CB, DeAngelis B, Frank O, Baker ER. Cobalamin (vitamin b12) and holotranscobalamin changes in plasma and liver tissue in alcoholics with liver disease. *A Coll of Nutr.* 2013 Jun; 17(3):235-238.

[6] Beattie AD, Sherlock S. Ascorbic acid deficiency in liver disease. *Gut.* 1976 Aug; 17:571-575.

[7] Bémeur C, Butterworth RF. Nutrition in the management of cirrhosis and its neurological complications. *J. Clin. Exp. Hepatol.* 2014 Jun; 4:141-150.

[8] Bode C, Bode JC. Effect of alcohol consumption on the gut. *Best Pract. Res. Clin. Gastroenterol.* 2003 Aug; 17(4):575-592.

[9] Bresci G, Parisi G, Banti S. Management of hepatic encephalopathy with oral zinc supplementation: a long-term treatment. *Eur. J. Med.* 1993 Aug-Sept; 2(7):414-416.

[10] Bujanda L. The effects of alcohol consumption upon the gastrointestinal tract. *Am. J. Gastroenterol.* 2000 Dec; 95:3374-3382.

[11] Clugston RD, Blaner WS. The adverse effects of alcohol on vitamin A metabolism. *Nutrition.* 2012 May; 4(5):356-371.

[12] Cook CC, Hallwood P, Thomson AD. B vitamin deficiency and neurophyschiatric syndromes in alcohol misuse. *Alcohol Alcohol.* 1998 Jul-Aug: 33(4),317-336.

[13] Day E, Bentham PW, Callaghan R, Kuruvilla T, George S. Thiamine for prevention and treatment of Wernicke-Korsakoff Syndrome in people

who abuse alcohol. *Cochrane Database Syst. Rev.* 2013 Jul, 7:CD004033.

[14] de la Maza MP, Petermann M, Bunout D, Hirsch S. Effects of long-term vitamin E supplementation in alcoholic cirrhosis. *J. Am. Coll. Nutr.* 1995 Apr; 14(2):192-196.

[15] De Marzio DH, Navarro VJ. Hepatotoxicity of cardiovascular and antidiabetic medications. Lipid lowering agents. In, Kaplowitz N, DeLeve LD, editors. Drug-induced liver disease. 3rd ed. Amsterdam: Elsevier; 2013. p. 519-540.

[16] DiCecco SR, Francisco-Ziller N. Nurition in alcoholic liver disease. *Nutr. Clin. Pract.* 2006 Jun; 21(3):245-254.

[17] Gilman AG, Rall TW, Nies AS, Taylor P. Goodman and Gilman's The Pharmacological Basis of Therapeutics. 8th ed. New York: Pergamon Press; 1990.

[18] González-Reimers E, Quintero-Platt G, Rodríguez-Rodríguez E, Martínez-Riera A, Alvisa-Negrin J, Santolaria-Fernández F. Bone changes in alcoholic liver disease. *World J. Hepatol.* 2015 May; 7(9):1258-1264.

[19] Griffith CM, Schenker S. The role of nutritional therapy in alcoholic liver disease. *Alcohol Res. Health.* 2006; 29(4):296-306.

[20] Gyamfi MA, Wan YJ. Pathogenesis of alcoholic liver disease: the role of nuclear receptors. *Exp. Biol. Med. (Maywood).* 2010 May; 235(5):547-560.

[21] Halsted CH, Villanueva JA, Devlin AM, Niemelä O, Parkkila S, Garrow TA, Wallock LM, Shigenaga MK, Melnyk S, James SJ. Folate deficiency disturbs hepatic methionine metabolism and promotes liver injury in ethanol-fed micropigs. *Proc. Natl. Acad. Sci. USA.* 2002 July; 99(15):10072-10077.

[22] Halsted CH, Villanueva JA, Devlin AM, Chandler CJ. Metabolic interactions of alcohol and folate. *J. Nutr.* 2002 Aug; 132(8 suppl):2367S-2372S.

[23] Institute of Medicine. Food and Nutrition Board. Dietary Reference Intakes: Thiamine, Riboflavin, Niacin, Vitamin B6, Folate, Vitamin B12, Panthothenic Acid, Biotin, and Choline. Washington, DC: National Academy Press; 1998.

[24] Institute of Medicine. Food and Nutrition Board. Dietary References Intakes: Vitamin C, Vitamin E, Selenium, and Carotenoids. Washington, DC: National Academy Press; 2000.

[25] Jacob E, Baker SJ, Herbert V. Vitamin B12-binding proteins. *Physiol. Rev.* 1980; 60(3):918-959.

[26] Kang JY, Zhou Z. Zinc prevention and treatment of alcoholic liver disease. *Mol. Aspects Med.* 2005 Aug-Oct; 26(4-5);391-404.

[27] Kharbanda KK. Nicotinic acid supplementation in the context of alcoholic liver injury: friend or foe? *Alcohol. Clin. Exp. Res.* 2014 July; 38(7):1829-1831.

[28] Lecomte E, Herbeth B, Pirollet P, Chancerelle Y, Arnaud J, Musse N, Paille F, Siest G, Artur Y. Effect of alcohol consumption on blood antioxidant nutrients and oxidative stress indicators. *Am. J. Clin. Nutr.* 1994 Aug; 60(2):255-261.

[29] Leevy CM, Baker H, Tenhove W, Frank O, Cherrick GR. B-complex vitamins in liver disease of the alcoholic. *Am. J. Clin. Nutr.* 1965 Apr;16:339-346.

[30] Li Q, Xie G, Zhang W, Zhong W, Sun X, Tan X, Sun X, Jia W, Zhou Z. Dietary nicotinic acid supplementation ameliorates chronic alcohol-induced fatty liver in rats. *Alcohol. Clin. Exp. Res.* 2014 July; 38(7):1982-1992.

[31] Lieber CS. Relationships between nutrition, alcohol use, and liver disease. *Alcohol Res. Health.* 2003;27(3):220-231.

[32] Mancinelli R, Ceccanti M. Biomarkers in alcohol misuse: their role in the prevention and detection of thiamine deficiency. *Alcohol Alcohol.* 2009 Mar-Apr; 44(2):177-182.

[33] Medici V, Halsted CH. Folate, alcohol, and liver disease. *Mol. Nutr. Food Res.* 2013 Apr; 57(4):596-606.

[34] Medici V, Peerson JM, Stabler SP, French SW, Gregory JF 3rd, Virata MC, Albanese A, Bowlus CL, Devaraj S, Panacek EA, Rahim N, Richards JR, Rossaro L, Halsted CH. Impaired homocysteine transsulfuration is an indicator of alcoholic liver disease. *J. Hepatol.* 2010 Sept; 53(3):551-557.

[35] Mezey E, Potter JJ, Rennie-Tankersley L, Caballeria J, Pares A. A randomized placebo controlled trial of vitamin E for alcoholic hepatitis. *J. Hepatol.* 2004 Jan; 40(1):40-46.

[36] Mohammad MK, Zhanxiang Z, Cave M, Barve A, McClain CJ. Zinc and liver disease. *Nutr. Clin. Pract.* 2012 Feb; 27(1):8-20.

[37] Muncie HL, Yasinian Y, Oge L. Outpatient management of alcohol withdrawal syndrome. *Am. Fam. Physician.* 2013 Nov; 88(9):589-595.

[38] Nagy LE. Molecular aspects of alcohol metabolism: transcription factors involved in early ethanol-induced liver injury. *Annu. Rev. Nutr.* 2004;24:55-78.

[39] Poikolainen K, Alho H. Magnesium treatment in alcoholics: a randomized clinical trial. *Subst. Abuse Treat Prev. Policy.* 2008 Jan;3:1.

[40] Prohit V, Russo D, Salin M. Role of iron in alcoholic liver disease: introduction and summary of symposium. *Alcohol.* 2003 Jun; 30(2):93-97.

[41] Rees E, Gowing LR. Supplementary thiamine is still important in alcohol dependence. *Alcohol. Alcohol.* 2013 Jan-Feb; 48(1):88-92.

[42] Rosenthal WS, Adham NF, Lopez R, Cooperman JM. Riboflavin deficiency in complicated chronic alcoholism. *Am. J. Clin. Nutr.* 1973 Aug; 26(8):858-860.

[43] Rossi RE, Conte D, Massironi S. Diagnosis and treatment of nutritional deficiencies in alcoholic liver disease: overview of available evidence and open issues. *Dig. Liver Dis.* 2015 Oct; 47(10):819-825.

[44] Santolaria F, González-Reimers E, Pérez-Manzano JL, Milena A, Gómez-Rodriguez MA, González-Rodriguez A, de la Vega MJ, Martínez-Riera A. Osteopenia assessed by body composition analysis is related to malnutrition in alcoholic patients. *Alcohol.* 2000 Nov; 20(3);147-157.

[45] Stickel F, Hoehn B, Schuppan D, Seitz HK. Review article: nutritional therapy in alcoholic liver disease. *Alliment Pharmacol. Ther.* 2003 Aug; 18(4):357-373.

[46] The Alpha-Tocopherol, Beta Carotene Cancer Prevention Study Group. The effect of vitamin E and beta carotene on the incidence of lung cancer and other cancers in male smokers. *N. Engl. J. Med.* 1994 Apr; 330(15):1029-1035.

[47] Thomson AD. Mechanisms of vitamin deficiency in chornic alcohol misusers and the development of the Wernicke-Korsakoff syndrome. *Alcohol Alcohol.* 2000 May-Jun; 35(1): 2-7.

[48] Thomson AD, Cook CCH, Touquet R, Henry JA. The royal college of physicians report on alcohol: guidelines for managing wernicke's encephalopathy in the accident and emergency department. *Alcohol Alcohol.* 2002 Nov-Dec; 37(6):513-521.

[49] Tillotson JA, Baker EM. An enzymatic measurement of riboflavin status in man. *Am. J. Clin. Nutr.* 1972 Apr; 25(4):425-431.

[50] Veitch RB. Lumeng L, Li TK. Vitamin B6 metabolism in chronic alcohol abuse. *J. Clin. Invest.* 1975 May; 55(5):1026-1032.

[51] Zhou Z, Wang L, Song Z, Saari JT, McClain CJ, Kang YJ. Zinc supplementation prevents alcoholic liver injury in mice through attenuation of oxidative stress. *Am. J. Pathol.* 2005 Jun; 166(6):1681-1690.

In: Alcohol and the Liver
Editor: Gerond Lake-Bakaar
ISBN: 978-1-63484-400-0

Chapter 6

LIVER TRANSPLANTATION FOR ALCOHOLIC LIVER DISEASE

Saikiran Kilaru[1], MD, and Michael P. Curry[2,*], MD

[1] Global Health Fellow and Hospitalist, Department of Medicine, Beth Israel Deaconess Medical Center, Boston, MA, US

[2] Director of Hepatology, Department of Medicine, Beth Israel Deaconess Medical Center, Boston, MA, US

ABSTRACT

Though initially controversial, liver transplantation (LT) currently plays a vital role in definitive treatment for alcoholic cirrhosis, and is now one of the most common indications. Data are emerging that LT for severe alcoholic hepatitis that is unresponsive to medical management may also play a role, though it is more controversial. The main concern in alcoholic patients is risk of relapse, and post-transplant interventions have been shown to reduce recidivism. Special considerations for patients transplanted for alcoholic liver disease center around post-transplant interventions to improve mortality, such as tobacco cessation and surveillance for malignancy.

---

[*] Corresponding author: Michael P Curry, MD; Director of Hepatology; 110 Francis Street, Suite 8E; Boston, MA 02215; mcurry@bidmc.harvard.edu; Tel: 617-632-1070; Fax 617-632-1065.

1. Introduction

Sixty-eight percent of Americans drink at least one alcoholic beverage per month, but only about 10% of all drinkers account for 50% of the total yearly alcohol consumption in the U.S. [1, 2]. Excessive alcohol consumption is the third leading preventable cause of death in the United States [3, 4]. The association between alcohol use and alcoholic liver disease is well documented in the literature, and chronic alcohol use can cause liver injury. Heavy alcohol consumption can lead to hepatic steatosis, alcoholic hepatitis, and cirrhosis. There is usually a sequential progression through these disease states, however they can also all occur at one time in the same patient as demonstrated by liver biopsy studies [5]. About 20 percent of alcoholics and heavy drinkers develop hepatic steatosis. A further 20% will develop biopsy proven alcoholic hepatitis, and about 10 percent to 15 percent of people with alcoholism will develop cirrhosis [6, 7].

Hepatic decompensation, traditionally defined as jaundice, ascites, variceal bleeding, and hepatic encephalopathy, is the harbinger of mortality in cirrhosis. Each manifestation has a varied risk of mortality. The rate of decompensation in patients with compensated cirrhosis is roughly 3-5% per year [8]. One-year mortality in compensated cirrhosis ranges between 1–3.4%, but in decompensated cirrhosis, the mortality rate is much higher at 20–57% [9-11]. Other modifying factors such as continued alcohol ingestion will affect mortality. The 5-year survival rate for cirrhotic patients who abstain from alcohol is 90% as compared to 70% in cirrhotics who continue drinking [7]. The prognosis is significantly worse for actively drinking patients with decompensated cirrhosis, with mortality rates of greater than 60% at 5 years [12].

Several models have been used to predict patient survival in patients with alcoholic liver cirrhosis as well as alcoholic hepatitis. Disease severity as assessed by the MELD (Model For End-Stage Liver Disease) score is related to mortality. The MELD score, initially developed to predict 90-day mortality in cirrhotic patients undergoing transjugular intrahepatic portosystemic shunts (TIPS), is a reliable and useful indicator of short-term mortality in patients with cirrhosis regardless of etiology [13, 14]. Higher MELD scores signify more severe disease, and MELD score has been shown to be superior to Child-Pugh Turcotte (CPT) score and Maddrey's discriminant function (DF) for predicting mortality in patients with alcoholic cirrhosis [15]. The 90-day predicted mortality in patients who have decompensated cirrhosis with a MELD score ≥30 is 90% [13, 16]. Without LT, prognosis in patients with end-stage alcoholic liver disease is decidedly poor, and LT is the only definitive treatment for these patients.

Scoring systems for alcoholic hepatitis also enable clinicians to assess severity and prognosis. Maddrey's DF, developed in 1978 and modified in 1993, is the first and most widely used independent predictor of mortality based on a multivariate analysis [17], and is the initial formula recommended by the AASLD to stratify the patient's severity of illness. The DF is frequently used to stratify which patients should be considered for pharmacological therapy with corticosteroids. Moreover the Lille model allows clinicians to determine which patients are unlikely to respond to treatment. Using this model, Louvet et al. found steroid-responsive patients had a 6-month survival rate of 85%, as compared to 25% survival in steroid-non-responders [18]. Similar to alcoholic cirrhosis, MELD has been to shown to be a better and more dynamic predictor of in-hospital mortality than DF and CPT [19, 20]. Patients with alcoholic hepatitis and a MELD score of 30 or greater have an estimated 90-day mortality of 62% or more, regardless of treatment [21]. Though some of the more benign symptoms can remit, continued jaundice or renal failure are more ominous and signify poor prognosis [22, 23]. Survival is significantly reduced in women and in the elderly and is adversely affected by the presence of severe liver injury, as well as progression to cirrhosis and continued alcohol use [24].

Recovery is influenced by abstinence, severity of illness, and initiation of appropriate treatment, the mainstay of which is corticosteroids [25]. Corticosteroids use in alcoholic hepatitis has been controversial, especially given the heterogeneity of disease in many clinical trials [26]. However, a number of meta-analyses demonstrate reduced mortality in well-selected patients (DF > 32) treated with corticosteroids [27]. A recent multi-center randomized control trial revealed that although prednisolone was associated with a non-significant reduction in 28-day mortality, multivariate analysis accounting for baseline determinants of prognosis showed a 39% reduction in the risk of death in patients treated with prednisone at 28 days. Despite this reduction in short-term mortality, there was no difference noted in overall and transplant free survival at 90 days and 1 year [28]. There are a significant number of patients with alcoholic hepatitis who fail to respond to medical therapy and have a high mortality. The optimal management of these patients needs further investigation and some authors suggest that LT may have a role in the care of these patients [18, 29].

2. LIVER TRANSPLANTATION FOR ALCOHOLIC CIRRHOSIS

In the early years of LT, the NIH consensus development conference predicted that few patients with alcoholic liver disease (ALD) would be appropriate LT candidates because of likely complex medical and psychosocial issues [30]. Concern centered on the view that this is a self-inflicted disease and that recurrent alcohol abuse would lead to poor outcomes and poor compliance with medical care and immunosuppression.

In 1991, the Health Care Financing Administration (now the Centers for Medicare & Medicaid Services) identified alcoholic cirrhosis as one of the conditions for which payment was covered for LT, but at the same time recommended a "significant" period of pre-transplant abstinence, as well as an acceptable social support system [31]. The minimal listing criteria established by the United Network for Organ Sharing (UNOS) in 1996 did not include an absolute need for a 6–month period of abstinence for LT, though a 1997 consensus conference of the American Association for the Study of Liver Diseases (AASLD) and American Society of Transplant (AST) concluded that there is a strong consensus for six months of abstinence and hence the "six month rule" emerged. The intention of the "six month rule" rests on three main objectives: to evaluate the patient's motivation and consequent risk for recidivism; to improve transplant outcome; and, most importantly, to allow patients with ALD a chance to recover spontaneously.

Though it is not an explicit UNOS requirement, a majority of the liver transplant programs in the United States and Europe either require a fixed period of abstinence (usually 6 months), or at least place value on established abstinence during the assessment when evaluating alcoholic patients for LT [32, 33].

Initial results of LT for alcoholic cirrhosis were quite poor with 20% survival at 3 years compared to 29% in patients with non-alcoholic cirrhosis [34]. However, Starzl et al. made the first convincing argument for LT for patients with alcoholic cirrhosis [35]. His group showed 73% survival at one year in a series of 41 ALD patients, and that only 3% of these patients relapsed. Following these results, many transplant centers gave more consideration to patients with ALD. Accordingly, the 1996 NIH workshop on LT for patients with ALD concluded that LT for alcoholic cirrhosis afforded good outcomes, while also concluding that relapse post-LT was lower if patients completed rehabilitation programs beforehand [1]. In the decade after this NIH workshop, there was a significant increase in the proportion (8.6%) of patients transplanted for ALD [36]. As a consequence of these results and the fact that there are genetic and environmental factors that account for ALD, alcoholic cirrhosis is currently the second most common indication for LT in the US.

The patient and graft–survival rate in patients with ALD is comparable, if not better, than that of patients with non–ALD [31]. Data from 2003 European Liver Transplant Registry (ELTR) showed that the 1- and 5-year survival rates of patients with alcoholic cirrhosis who underwent LT to be 81% and 72%, respectively, which was identical to survival rates for patients transplanted for viral cirrhosis [37]. Subsequent data from the ELTR and the United States showed slightly improved survival for patients transplanted for ALD in comparison to patients transplanted for viral etiologies, and has also showed significantly better overall unadjusted survival in comparison to patients transplanted for cryptogenic cirrhosis [36, 38]. Patients who were transplanted for ALD also have decreased incidence of acute cellular rejection, and patients transplanted for ALD and hepatitis C virus (HCV) have similar incidence of acute rejection compared to patients transplanted for non-alcoholic liver disease [36, 39]. Finally, the incidence of re-transplantation in patients with ALD is less compared to patients transplanted for other etiologies [39].

The physical and psychological outcomes for ALD patients after LT appear similar to those of non–ALD patients [40]. In patients who experience relapse, quality of life outcomes are noted to be lower [41]. Though fewer patients with ALD are employed in comparison to patients without ALD prior to transplant, there is no difference in rates of employment post-transplantation [42].

3. Liver Transplantation for Alcoholic Hepatitis

The serious risk of early death in patients with severe alcoholic hepatitis who fail to respond to medical therapy represents a significant challenge as most of these patients have recent heavy alcohol ingestion prior to presentation and no significant periods of abstinence. Controversy surrounding the six-month rule is part of a larger debate surrounding transplantation in acute alcoholic hepatitis. There are several current limitations to being listed for transplant as an active drinker. A patient with severe symptomatic alcoholic hepatitis would likely have difficulty undergoing an extensive psychological evaluation. There is no time period in which a patient can be referred for treatment of addiction in the acute setting [43]. Public support can be scarce, especially in light of controversial transplantation of celebrities, which resulted in visible recidivism. In addition, with the current MELD-based allocation system, patients with acute alcoholic hepatitis and liver failure would receive a high degree of priority on the transplant waiting list. This is important, because public support drives donor registry, and in the current climate of organ shortage, this could impact organ donation rates.

Currently, while prospective data are limited, and public support is also similarly limited, transplantation for alcoholic hepatitis is controversial. Most transplant programs in the United States currently regard acute alcoholic hepatitis as a contraindication to LT. In contrast, the European Association for Study of the Liver (EASL) therapeutic algorithm for management of alcoholic hepatitis allows for consideration of early LT as a treatment option in selected patients with alcoholic hepatitis [44]. Accordingly, data are limited regarding outcomes of LT for patients with acute alcoholic hepatitis, but some data on outcomes of early LT are accumulating from Europe and the U.S. [29, 45].

A case series from Pittsburgh published in 1997 identified 9 patients with acute severe alcoholic hepatitis with DF scores of >32 who had undergone LT. This constituted 1.9% of all transplants performed at this center. Four of the 9 patients were actively drinking at the time of admission and all patients were CPT class C. Explant liver tissue on all patients demonstrated mixed micro- and macro-vesicular steatosis, Mallory's hyaline and polymorphonuclear infiltrates consistent with alcoholic hepatitis. Kaplan-Meier survival analysis of patients receiving LT for acute alcoholic hepatitis with a DF > 32, a DF of < 32 and for alcohol cirrhosis did not show a difference in patient survival [46].

A larger prospective study published by Mathurin et al. from multiple centers in France and Brussels of early LT in patients with severe alcoholic hepatitis who failed steroid therapy with a median Lille score of 0.88 shows excellent outcomes [29]. The survival at 6 months post-transplantation was 77%, which is comparable to the results of LT for other acute indications [47]. Survival at 6 months was significantly better for transplant recipients at 77% as compared to that of the control group at 23%. Another success of this study was the low rate of relapse: at 2-3 years of follow-up, relapse rate post-LT was 11%. Some of this success of this study may be related to the rigorous selection process; some of the centers selected less than 2% of the recruited pool of patients with severe alcoholic hepatitis for LT. The selection process in this study was particularly involved. Only patients with their first liver-decompensating event were considered (patients with recent jaundice or gastrointestinal hemorrhage were included, but not any other decompensating event); patients had to be deemed non-responders to medical therapy (DF > 32 and Lille score of 0.45 or more after 7 days of medical therapy, or a continuous increase in MELD score); they had to have close supportive family members who could be involved in the process; finally, patients with severe coexisting or psychiatric disorders were not included, even if these disorders were proven to be stably managed, because of the brisk timing of the selection process. Eligible patients underwent a selection process consisting of several meetings with four sequential medical and surgical teams, all of whom had to be in agreement that the patient was a suitable candidate for LT. It is possible that patients who were selected could have had different socioeconomic backgrounds and demographics from those who were not selected, though only age and sex were reported in the baseline characteristics. An accompanying editorial points out that an accurate objective tool to predict the risk of recidivism is needed to allow equitable selection of candidates [48]. This study concluded that early LT is likely viable in a carefully selected group of patients with severe alcoholic hepatitis, with acceptable short-term survival and low rates of post-transplant alcohol relapse.

In two other retrospective studies, a small cohort of patients transplanted for alcoholic hepatitis had similar patient and graft survival rates as did those in a matched control population of patients transplanted for alcoholic cirrhosis [45, 49]. Using the United Network for Organ Sharing (UNOS) database, one study looked at 55 patients who underwent LT for alcoholic hepatitis and compared them to 165 matched patients transplanted for alcoholic cirrhosis. At 1, 3 and 5 years, there were no differences in graft and patient survival. Even though more patients transplanted for alcoholic hepatitis had HCV, after controlling for this, outcomes were still similar. Finally, they also compared groups based on explant diagnosis of alcoholic hepatitis and alcoholic cirrhosis, and outcomes were again similar [45]. Another study based on explant diagnosis compared patients with and without histological evidence of acute alcoholic hepatitis with patients transplanted for non-ALD. Patient and graft survival between patients with histologic evidence of alcoholic hepatitis and bland alcoholic cirrhosis were similar. The patients with histologic proven alcoholic hepatitis and those with bland alcoholic cirrhosis had no differences in post-transplantation relapse (roughly 16%), and there was no difference in graft loss or survival compared with controls [49].

Future prospective studies are needed to explore the specifics of post-transplant outcomes, including intermediate- and longer-term survival, long-term relapse rates, and ethical implications of stringent selection for alcoholic hepatitis. In addition, consideration should be taken to determine the effect of transplanting patients with acute alcoholic hepatitis on public perception and on organ donation rates.

4. Timing of Transplantation

Timing of transplantation involves pre-transplantation consideration for referral, as well as consideration of the natural history of alcoholic cirrhosis, alcoholic hepatitis, and alcoholism itself. Part of the challenge of transplantation for alcoholic liver disease lies antecedent to selection. Though LT for alcoholic cirrhosis has been well established as a viable and critical treatment option, challenges remain in obtaining access. Surveys of both primary care physicians and gastroenterologists show that they are less likely to prioritize LT for alcoholic liver disease [50].

A retrospective VA study of 199 potential LT candidates with end-stage alcoholic liver disease, showed that only 21% were recommended for referral, and only 8% actually underwent transplant evaluation. The significant negative independent determinants for discussion of LT in this study were older age, alcoholic liver disease, and black race. It is conceivable that many patients could have had contraindications, but these were inferred and not routinely documented, but a small significant proportion (7%) had no recorded evidence of contraindications at all [51]. It is difficult to know whether this can be generalized to other transplant centers, as the transplant referral process through the VA is centralized, and evaluation can only be performed at 4 VA transplant centers in the U.S.

The minimal criteria for placement on the LT waiting list, formulated in 1997, requires patients to have hepatic decompensation as determined by the CPT score, which must be greater than or equal to 7 [52]. It is important to note that patients with Child-Pugh class B alcoholic cirrhosis can spontaneously improve and have meaningful survival with standard medical management and thus immediate listing for transplant has been shown not to improve survival or prevent liver-related mortality in these patients [53]. This study suggests that some patients with Child-Pugh stage B alcoholic cirrhosis do not need to be immediate listed for LT, especially when alcohol withdrawal maybe associated with recovery of liver function, particularly when the CPT score is less than 8. This supports giving priority for organ allocation to sicker patients, and is supported by previous data which showed that patients with the most severe disease ALD (Child-Pugh stage C) benefitted most from LT, with higher 1- and 5-year survival when compared to patients at lower risk, i.e., Child-Pugh stage A or B [54].

5. Outcomes Following Relapse after Liver Transplantation

In most cases, alcohol relapse does not influence 1-year and 5-year survival rates after LT for alcoholic cirrhosis [55-57]. As such, in short and medium term time periods, relapse has minimal effect on survival. Pageaux et al. also report that in the intermediate term, recidivism did not affect survival and compliance with post-transplant immunosuppressive regimen [57]. However, in analyses of long-term survival after LT for alcoholic cirrhosis, Cuadrado et al. reported a significantly worse survival in patients with harmful alcohol relapse after LT [58]. This study also simultaneously showed that the most frequent causes of death in patients with alcohol relapse after LT were cardiovascular events and malignancies. Similarly, Dumortier et al. showed that at 10 years, other target-organ damage of both alcohol and tobacco contributed to reduced survival, especially in the form of malignancy, but that alcohol relapse was not a significant prognostic factor for survival [59].

Furthermore, there are decidedly different levels of alcohol consumption patterns after LT. Whereas most transplant centers consider any alcohol consumption a relapse, many addiction specialists feel that a slip (brief, minor lapse followed by abstinence) is much more minor than true relapse to abusive drinking. Because the definition of relapse varies, relapse rates reported in the literature range from 7% to 95% [55, 57].

These different levels of consumption lead to different prognoses after LT. Recently, the emphasis on post-transplant alcohol use has shifted to focus more on the pattern of use as opposed to the frequency [60]. It appears that some patients are predisposed to binge drinking. In a prospective study of 167 post-LT patients, 20% of those who relapsed had a binge episode, and all of them drank more than 6 drinks during this episode [61]. Pfitzmann et al. showed that survival rates of patients transplanted for ALD who resumed abusive drinking were significantly lower than survival rates of abstinent patients or patients with minor lapses [62]. It is important to note that this study differentiated patients based on patterns of drinking, whereas prior studies did not. In contrast to prior studies, they showed that the majority of deaths in patients who resumed abusive drinking after LT were due to recurrent alcoholic liver disease, whereas abstinent patients predominantly died of malignant tumors, infections, and cardiovascular disease. They also showed that patients who resumed abusive drinking had five and ten-year survival rates of 69.5% and 20.1% respectively, compared to 90.3% and 81.5% in abstinent patients.

For this reason, it is standard to evaluate patients pre-transplant with a multidisciplinary team that includes an addiction specialist. Interestingly, transplant centers have shown that their relapse rate dropped from 32% to 13% after an addiction psychologist became a permanent fixture of pre-transplant evaluation and post-transplant follow-up [47]. As such, there is evidence that more than solely relying on psychosocial selection, specific pre- and post-transplantation involvement and counseling can minimize risk of relapse. Successful transplantation in patients with alcoholic cirrhosis relies heavily on careful selection of candidates. Selection criteria are not standardized across UNOS centers, but apart from medical and surgical features, they generally center on sobriety and psychosocial factors. The six-month rule for abstinence, discussed elsewhere, is widely debated but centered on the principle that post-transplant compliance and recidivism can be inferred by a patient's ability to remain abstinent. Patients are also evaluated on their level of functioning, social support and demonstration of insight.

Predicting recidivism is notoriously difficult. There are conflicting data on whether reported prognosticators are truly predictive of lasting abstinence. DiMartini et al. reported in a univariate model that at five years, predictors of alcohol use were pre-transplant length of sobriety, diagnosis of alcohol dependence, history of other substance use, and prior alcohol rehabilitation [61]. Multivariate analysis showed that pre-transplant sobriety of less than 6 months, absence of a companion in life, presence of young children, and a predicted poor psychosomatic prognosis were associated with an increased risk of recurrent alcohol consumption, though this study could have been biased due to observational bias and recall bias [62].

The six-month rule remains controversial. In fact Vaillant reported that five years of sobriety was the most powerful marker of future abstinence in the long-term [63]. Though data from single-center, retrospective trials have shown that duration of abstinence is a predictor of recidivism [61, 64, 65], others have concluded that the length of pre-transplant abstinence is a poor predictor of relapse [66, 67]. In general, studies of recidivism after LT are plagued with generalizability issues: they are fraught with differences in definitions of relapse and in methods of follow up and self-reporting. In clinical practice, self-report is undermined by the patient's conflict of interest. Other objective markers, such as liver histology suggesting acute alcoholic hepatitis, are also not predictive of relapse [49]. For this reason, psychiatric and psychosocial evaluation by a multi-disciplinary team that includes an addiction specialist in the pre-transplant period is standard.

6. Post-Transplantation Care

Patients transplanted for ALD have a unique set of needs after LT. Performing a comprehensive pre-transplant evaluation in conjunction with post-transplant follow-up with these specialists is integral to prevention and management of relapse. The idea is that these specialists can identify patients at risk or who have already relapsed and intervene [68]. Burra and Lucey state that identifying patients at higher risk of relapse is the biggest challenge in the post-transplant period [69].

Though pre-transplant substance abuse treatment is standard at most transplant programs, post-transplant treatment is not universal. A study of 118 patients undergoing LT and combined liver kidney transplantation (LKT) found that those who received substance abuse treatment before and after LT had significantly lower recidivism rates (16%) than patients who received no treatment (41%) or only pre-transplant treatment (45%) [70]. Treatment is likely best accomplished with addiction specialists on the team, especially given that medications such as naltrexone, used in the pharmacologic treatment of alcohol dependence, can be hepatotoxic. Whether patients who attend more intensive substance abuse treatment have lower rates of relapse has not been studied.

Tobacco use and alcoholism go hand-in-hand, and the use of tobacco is a substantial risk factor for post-transplant morbidity and mortality. A VA study revealed that 90% of alcoholics also smoke [71]. A single center survey study found that 60% of LT recipients had a lifetime history of tobacco use, with 15% smoking post-LT. Just as concerning was the 20% relapse relate in patients who had quit tobacco prior to LT [72]. In addition, the patients that resume smoking post-LT exhibit detrimental behaviors, starting early post-transplant, increasing their consumption over time, and quickly becoming tobacco dependent [73].

Active smoking (independent of alcohol relapse) is one of the major risk factors for long-term morbidity and mortality from cardiovascular complications or malignancy in ALD patients post-transplant [74]. The carcinogenic effects of alcohol and tobacco are likely compounded by post-LT immunosuppression. Herrero et al. showed that patients who previously smoked and continued after LT had a hazard ratio of approximately 20 for the development of neoplasms associated with tobacco, much higher than in patients who quit [75]. In terms of transplant-specific mortality, patients with a history of smoking had a higher rate of post-LT vascular complications (thrombosis, stenosis), which require urgent intervention and often re-transplantation, with significant subsequent morbidity and mortality [76]. Those who quit smoking 2 years prior to LT had a lower risk. Because of the aforementioned risk for worsened mortality and morbidity in association with tobacco abuse, alcohol relapse should not be the sole focus in the peri-transplant period. Pre- and post-LT follow-up should also include tobacco use surveillance and cessation counseling.

Patients who undergo transplant for ALD have a higher rate of cancers (especially of the aerodigestive tract) in comparison to those who undergo LT for non-alcohol related conditions [77, 78]. These malignancies are a major cause of illness and death late after LT [79]. Accordingly, many transplant centers are developing protocols for tumor surveillance; early results have shown improved survival in patients who were enrolled in these surveillance protocols [80, 81].

Conclusion

Alcoholic cirrhosis is an accepted indication for LT with good patient and graft outcomes. Transplantation for alcoholic hepatitis is controversial, but in carefully selected patients, it may have a role. It requires further investigation with prospective data, as well as examining the bias and reproducibility of strict selection criteria. Though recidivism is a concern, particularly relapse to abusive or heavy drinking, post-transplant counseling for alcohol and tobacco abstinence is important and can play an ameliorative role. The post-transplant period is also critical for tobacco abstinence counseling. Ongoing surveillance for malignancy, and preventive care for cardiovascular events needed.

REFERENCES

[1] Hoofnagle JH, Kresina T, Fuller RK, Lake JR, Lucey MR, Sorrell MF, et al. Liver transplantation for alcoholic liver disease: executive statement and recommendations. Summary of a National Institutes of Health workshop held December 6-7, 1996, Bethesda, Maryland. Liver transplantation and surgery: official publication of the American Association for the Study of Liver Diseases and the International Liver Transplantation Society. 1997;3(3):347-50.

[2] Li TK. Research direction. Liver transplantation and surgery: official publication of the American Association for the Study of Liver Diseases and the International Liver Transplantation Society. 1997;3(3):296-9.

[3] Centers for Disease C, Prevention. Alcohol-attributable deaths and years of potential life lost--United States, 2001. MMWR Morbidity and mortality weekly report. 2004;53(37):866-70.

[4] Mokdad AH, Marks JS, Stroup DF, Gerberding JL. Actual causes of death in the United States, 2000. *JAMA*. 2004;291(10):1238-45.

[5] Kirsch RE, Robson S, Trey C. Diagnosis and management of liver disease. 1st ed. London; New York: Chapman & Hall Medical; 1995. xv, 327 p., 4 p. of plates. p.

[6] Naveau S, Giraud V, Borotto E, Aubert A, Capron F, Chaput JC. Excess weight risk factor for alcoholic liver disease. *Hepatology*. 1997;25(1):108-11.

[7] Mann RE, Smart RG, Govoni R. The epidemiology of alcoholic liver disease. Alcohol research & health: *The journal of the National Institute on Alcohol Abuse and Alcoholism*. 2003;27(3):209-19.

[8] Fleming KM, Aithal GP, Card TR, West J. The rate of decompensation and clinical progression of disease in people with cirrhosis: a cohort study. *Alimentary pharmacology & therapeutics*. 2010;32(11-12):1343-50.

[9] D'Amico G, Garcia-Tsao G, Pagliaro L. Natural history and prognostic indicators of survival in cirrhosis: a systematic review of 118 studies. *Journal of hepatology*. 2006;44(1):217-31.

[10] D'Amico G, Morabito A, Pagliaro L, Marubini E. Survival and prognostic indicators in compensated and decompensated cirrhosis. *Digestive diseases and sciences*. 1986;31(5):468-75.

[11] de Franchis R. Evolving consensus in portal hypertension. Report of the Baveno IV consensus workshop on methodology of diagnosis and

therapy in portal hypertension. *Journal of hepatology*. 2005;43(1):167-76.

[12] Dugum M, McCullough A. Diagnosis and Management of Alcoholic Liver Disease. *Journal of clinical and translational hepatology*. 2015;3(2):109-16.

[13] Kamath PS, Wiesner RH, Malinchoc M, Kremers W, Therneau TM, Kosberg CL, et al. A model to predict survival in patients with end-stage liver disease. *Hepatology*. 2001;33(2):464-70.

[14] Mukerji AN, Patel V, Jain A. Improving survival in decompensated cirrhosis. *International journal of hepatology*. 2012;2012:318627.

[15] Xie YD, Feng B, Gao Y, Wei L. Characteristics of alcoholic liver disease and predictive factors for mortality of patients with alcoholic cirrhosis. Hepatobiliary & pancreatic diseases international: HBPD INT. 2013;12(6):594-601.

[16] Said A, Williams J, Holden J, Remington P, Gangnon R, Musat A, et al. Model for end stage liver disease score predicts mortality across a broad spectrum of liver disease. *Journal of hepatology*. 2004;40(6):897-903.

[17] Monsanto P, Almeida N, Lrias C, Pina JE, Sofia C. Evaluation of MELD score and Maddrey discriminant function for mortality prediction in patients with alcoholic hepatitis. *Hepato-gastroenterology*. 2013;60(125):1089-94.

[18] Louvet A, Naveau S, Abdelnour M, Ramond MJ, Diaz E, Fartoux L, et al. The Lille model: a new tool for therapeutic strategy in patients with severe alcoholic hepatitis treated with steroids. *Hepatology*. 2007;45(6):1348-54.

[19] Sheth M, Riggs M, Patel T. Utility of the Mayo End-Stage Liver Disease (MELD) score in assessing prognosis of patients with alcoholic hepatitis. *BMC gastroenterology*. 2002;2:2.

[20] Srikureja W, Kyulo NL, Runyon BA, Hu KQ. MELD score is a better prognostic model than Child-Turcotte-Pugh score or Discriminant Function score in patients with alcoholic hepatitis. *Journal of hepatology*. 2005;42(5):700-6.

[21] Dunn W, Jamil LH, Brown LS, Wiesner RH, Kim WR, Menon KV, et al. MELD accurately predicts mortality in patients with alcoholic hepatitis. *Hepatology*. 2005;41(2):353-8.

[22] Mathurin P, Abdelnour M, Ramond MJ, Carbonell N, Fartoux L, Serfaty L, et al. Early change in bilirubin levels is an important prognostic factor in severe alcoholic hepatitis treated with prednisolone. *Hepatology*. 2003;38(6):1363-9.

[23] Mutimer DJ, Burra P, Neuberger JM, Hubscher S, Buckels JA, Mayer AD, et al. Managing severe alcoholic hepatitis complicated by renal failure. *The Quarterly journal of medicine.* 1993;86(10):649-56.
[24] Morgan MY. The prognosis and outcome of alcoholic liver disease. *Alcohol and alcoholism.* 1994;2:335-43.
[25] Lucey MR, Mathurin P, Morgan TR. Alcoholic hepatitis. *The New England journal of medicine.* 2009;360(26):2758-69.
[26] Mathurin P, Lucey MR. Management of alcoholic hepatitis. *Journal of hepatology.* 2012;56 Suppl 1:S39-45.
[27] Rambaldi A, Saconato HH, Christensen E, Thorlund K, Wetterslev J, Gluud C. Systematic review: glucocorticosteroids for alcoholic hepatitis--a Cochrane Hepato-Biliary Group systematic review with meta-analyses and trial sequential analyses of randomized clinical trials. *Alimentary pharmacology & therapeutics.* 2008;27(12):1167-78.
[28] Thursz MR, Richardson P, Allison M, Austin A, Bowers M, Day CP, et al. Prednisolone or pentoxifylline for alcoholic hepatitis. *The New England journal of medicine.* 2015;372(17):1619-28.
[29] Mathurin P, Moreno C, Samuel D, Dumortier J, Salleron J, Durand F, et al. Early liver transplantation for severe alcoholic hepatitis. *The New England journal of medicine.* 2011;365(19):1790-800.
[30] National Institutes of Health Consensus Development Conference Statement: liver transplantation--June 20-23, 1983. *Hepatology.* 1984;4(1 Suppl):107S-10S.
[31] Anantharaju A, Van Thiel DH. Liver transplantation for alcoholic liver disease. Alcohol research & health: the journal of the National Institute on Alcohol Abuse and Alcoholism. 2003;27(3):257-68.
[32] Beresford TP, Everson GT. Liver transplantation for alcoholic liver disease: bias, beliefs, 6-month rule, and relapse--but where are the data? Liver transplantation: official publication of the American Association for the Study of Liver Diseases and the International Liver Transplantation Society. 2000;6(6):777-8.
[33] Everhart JE, Beresford TP. Liver transplantation for alcoholic liver disease: a survey of transplantation programs in the United States. Liver transplantation and surgery: official publication of the American Association for the Study of Liver Diseases and the International Liver Transplantation Society. 1997;3(3):220-6.
[34] Scharschmidt BF. Human liver transplantation: analysis of data on 540 patients from four centers. *Hepatology.* 1984;4(1 Suppl):95S-101S.

[35] Starzl TE, Van Thiel D, Tzakis AG, Iwatsuki S, Todo S, Marsh JW, et al. Orthotopic liver transplantation for alcoholic cirrhosis. *JAMA*. 1988;260(17):2542-4.

[36] Burra P, Senzolo M, Adam R, Delvart V, Karam V, Germani G, et al. Liver transplantation for alcoholic liver disease in Europe: a study from the ELTR (European Liver Transplant Registry). American journal of transplantation: official journal of the American Society of *Transplantation and the American Society of Transplant Surgeons*. 2010;10(1):138-48.

[37] Adam R, McMaster P, O'Grady JG, Castaing D, Klempnauer JL, Jamieson N, et al. Evolution of liver transplantation in Europe: report of the European Liver Transplant Registry. Liver transplantation: official publication of the American Association for the Study of Liver Diseases and the International Liver Transplantation Society. 2003;9(12):1231-43.

[38] Lucey MR, Schaubel DE, Guidinger MK, Tome S, Merion RM. Effect of alcoholic liver disease and hepatitis C infection on waiting list and posttransplant mortality and transplant survival benefit. *Hepatology*. 2009;50(2):400-6.

[39] Wiesner RH, Lombardero M, Lake JR, Everhart J, Detre KM. Liver transplantation for end-stage alcoholic liver disease: an assessment of outcomes. Liver transplantation and surgery: official publication of the American Association for the Study of Liver Diseases and the International Liver Transplantation Society. 1997;3(3):231-9.

[40] Pereira SP, Howard LM, Muiesan P, Rela M, Heaton N, Williams R. Quality of life after liver transplantation for alcoholic liver disease. Liver transplantation: official publication of the American Association for the Study of Liver Diseases and the International Liver Transplantation Society. 2000;6(6):762-8.

[41] Coffman KL, Hoffman A, Sher L, Rojter S, Vierling J, Makowka L. Treatment of the postoperative alcoholic liver transplant recipient with other addictions. Liver transplantation and surgery: official publication of the American Association for the Study of Liver Diseases and the International Liver Transplantation Society. 1997;3(3):322-7.

[42] Bravata DM, Keeffe EB. Quality of life and employment after liver transplantation. Liver transplantation: official publication of the American Association for the Study of Liver Diseases and the International Liver Transplantation Society. 2001;7(11 Suppl 1):S119-23.

[43] Berlakovich GA. Challenges in transplantation for alcoholic liver disease. *World journal of gastroenterology*. 2014;20(25):8033-9.
[44] European Association for the Study of L. EASL clinical practical guidelines: management of alcoholic liver disease. *Journal of hepatology*. 2012;57(2):399-420.
[45] Singal AK, Bashar H, Anand BS, Jampana SC, Singal V, Kuo YF. Outcomes after liver transplantation for alcoholic hepatitis are similar to alcoholic cirrhosis: exploratory analysis from the UNOS database. *Hepatology*. 2012;55(5):1398-405.
[46] Shakil AO, Pinna A, Demetris J, Lee RG, Fung JJ, Rakela J. Survival and quality of life after liver transplantation for acute alcoholic hepatitis. Liver transplantation and surgery: official publication of the American Association for the Study of Liver Diseases and the International Liver Transplantation Society. 1997;3(3):240-4.
[47] Berlakovich GA, Langer F, Freundorfer E, Windhager T, Rockenschaub S, Sporn E, et al. General compliance after liver transplantation for alcoholic cirrhosis. *Transplant international: official journal of the European Society for Organ Transplantation*. 2000;13(2):129-35.
[48] Brown RS, Jr. Transplantation for alcoholic hepatitis--time to rethink the 6-month "rule." *The New England journal of medicine*. 2011; 365(19):1836-8.
[49] Wells JT, Said A, Agni R, Tome S, Hughes S, Dureja P, et al. The impact of acute alcoholic hepatitis in the explanted recipient liver on outcome after liver transplantation. Liver transplantation: official publication of the American Association for the Study of Liver Diseases and the International Liver Transplantation Society. 2007;13(12):1728-35.
[50] Neuberger J, Adams D, MacMaster P, Maidment A, Speed M. Assessing priorities for allocation of donor liver grafts: survey of public and clinicians. *BMJ*. 1998;317(7152):172-5.
[51] Julapalli VR, Kramer JR, El-Serag HB, American Association for the Study of Liver D. Evaluation for liver transplantation: adherence to AASLD referral guidelines in a large Veterans Affairs center. Liver transplantation: official publication of the American Association for the Study of Liver Diseases and the International Liver Transplantation Society. 2005;11(11):1370-8.
[52] Lucey MR, Brown KA, Everson GT, Fung JJ, Gish R, Keeffe EB, et al. Minimal criteria for placement of adults on the liver transplant waiting list: a report of a national conference organized by the American Society

of Transplant Physicians and the American Association for the Study of Liver Diseases. Liver transplantation and surgery: official publication of the American Association for the Study of Liver Diseases and the International Liver Transplantation Society. 1997;3(6):628-37.

[53] Vanlemmens C, Di Martino V, Milan C, Messner M, Minello A, Duvoux C, et al. Immediate listing for liver transplantation versus standard care for Child-Pugh stage B alcoholic cirrhosis: a randomized trial. *Annals of internal medicine*. 2009;150(3):153-61.

[54] Poynard T, Naveau S, Doffoel M, Boudjema K, Vanlemmens C, Mantion G, et al. Evaluation of efficacy of liver transplantation in alcoholic cirrhosis using matched and simulated controls: 5-year survival. Multi-centre group. *Journal of hepatology*. 1999;30(6):1130-7.

[55] Bjornsson E, Olsson J, Rydell A, Fredriksson K, Eriksson C, Sjoberg C, et al. Long-term follow-up of patients with alcoholic liver disease after liver transplantation in Sweden: impact of structured management on recidivism. *Scandinavian journal of gastroenterology*. 2005;40(2):206-16.

[56] Mackie J, Groves K, Hoyle A, Garcia C, Garcia R, Gunson B, et al. Orthotopic liver transplantation for alcoholic liver disease: a retrospective analysis of survival, recidivism, and risk factors predisposing to recidivism. Liver transplantation: official publication of the American Association for the Study of Liver Diseases and the International Liver Transplantation Society. 2001;7(5):418-27.

[57] Pageaux GP, Michel J, Coste V, Perney P, Possoz P, Perrigault PF, et al. Alcoholic cirrhosis is a good indication for liver transplantation, even for cases of recidivism. *GUT*. 1999;45(3):421-6.

[58] Cuadrado A, Fabrega E, Casafont F, Pons-Romero F. Alcohol recidivism impairs long-term patient survival after orthotopic liver transplantation for alcoholic liver disease. Liver transplantation: official publication of the American Association for the Study of Liver Diseases and the International Liver Transplantation Society. 2005;11(4):420-6.

[59] Dumortier J, Guillaud O, Adham M, Boucaud C, Delafosse B, Bouffard Y, et al. Negative impact of de novo malignancies rather than alcohol relapse on survival after liver transplantation for alcoholic cirrhosis: a retrospective analysis of 305 patients in a single center. *The American journal of gastroenterology*. 2007;102(5):1032-41.

[60] Fuller RK. Definition and diagnosis of relapse to drinking. Liver transplantation and surgery: official publication of the American

Association for the Study of Liver Diseases and the International Liver Transplantation Society. 1997;3(3):258-62.

[61] DiMartini A, Day N, Dew MA, Javed L, Fitzgerald MG, Jain A, et al. Alcohol consumption patterns and predictors of use following liver transplantation for alcoholic liver disease. Liver transplantation: official publication of the American Association for the Study of Liver Diseases and the International Liver Transplantation Society. 2006;12(5):813-20.

[62] Pfitzmann R, Schwenzer J, Rayes N, Seehofer D, Neuhaus R, Nussler NC. Long-term survival and predictors of relapse after orthotopic liver transplantation for alcoholic liver disease. Liver transplantation: official publication of the American Association for the Study of Liver Diseases and the International Liver Transplantation Society. 2007;13(2):197-205.

[63] Vaillant GE. A 60-year follow-up of alcoholic men. *Addiction.* 2003;98(8):1043-51.

[64] Karim Z, Intaraprasong P, Scudamore CH, Erb SR, Soos JG, Cheung E, et al. Predictors of relapse to significant alcohol drinking after liver transplantation. Canadian journal of gastroenterology. *Journal canadien de gastroenterologie.* 2010;24(4):245-50.

[65] Perney P, Bismuth M, Sigaud H, Picot MC, Jacquet E, Puche P, et al. Are preoperative patterns of alcohol consumption predictive of relapse after liver transplantation for alcoholic liver disease? Transplant international: official journal of the European Society for Organ Transplantation. 2005;18(11):1292-7.

[66] Foster PF, Fabrega F, Karademir S, Sankary HN, Mital D, Williams JW. Prediction of abstinence from ethanol in alcoholic recipients following liver transplantation. *Hepatology.* 1997;25(6):1469-77.

[67] Kelly M, Chick J, Gribble R, Gleeson M, Holton M, Winstanley J, et al. Predictors of relapse to harmful alcohol after orthotopic liver transplantation. *Alcohol Alcohol.* 2006;41(3):278-83.

[68] Iruzubieta P, Crespo J, Fabrega E. Long-term survival after liver transplantation for alcoholic liver disease. *World journal of gastroenterology.* 2013;19(48):9198-208.

[69] Burra P, Lucey MR. Liver transplantation in alcoholic patients. Transplant international: official journal of the European Society for Organ Transplantation. 2005;18(5):491-8.

[70] Rodrigue JR, Hanto DW, Curry MP. Substance abuse treatment and its association with relapse to alcohol use after liver transplantation. Liver transplantation: official publication of the American Association for the

Study of Liver Diseases and the International Liver Transplantation Society. 2013;19(12):1387-95.

[71] Burling TA, Ziff DC. Tobacco smoking: a comparison between alcohol and drug abuse inpatients. *Addictive behaviors*. 1988;13(2):185-90.

[72] Ehlers SL, Rodrigue JR, Widows MR, Reed AI, Nelson DR. Tobacco use before and after liver transplantation: a single center survey and implications for clinical practice and research. Liver transplantation: official publication of the American Association for the Study of Liver Diseases and the International Liver Transplantation Society. 2004;10(3):412-7.

[73] DiMartini A, Javed L, Russell S, Dew MA, Fitzgerald MG, Jain A, et al. Tobacco use following liver transplantation for alcoholic liver disease: an underestimated problem. Liver transplantation: official publication of the American Association for the Study of Liver Diseases and the International Liver Transplantation Society. 2005;11(6):679-83.

[74] Kotlyar DS, Burke A, Campbell MS, Weinrieb RM. A critical review of candidacy for orthotopic liver transplantation in alcoholic liver disease. *The American journal of gastroenterology*. 2008;103(3):734-43; quiz 44.

[75] Herrero JI, Pardo F, D'Avola D, Alegre F, Rotellar F, Inarrairaegui M, et al. Risk factors of lung, head and neck, esophageal, and kidney and urinary tract carcinomas after liver transplantation: the effect of smoking withdrawal. Liver transplantation: official publication of the American Association for the Study of Liver Diseases and the International Liver Transplantation Society. 2011;17(4):402-8.

[76] Pungpapong S, Manzarbeitia C, Ortiz J, Reich DJ, Araya V, Rothstein KD, et al. Cigarette smoking is associated with an increased incidence of vascular complications after liver transplantation. Liver transplantation: official publication of the American Association for the Study of Liver Diseases and the International Liver Transplantation Society. 2002;8(7):582-7.

[77] Pruthi J, Medkiff KA, Esrason KT, Donovan JA, Yoshida EM, Erb SR, et al. Analysis of causes of death in liver transplant recipients who survived more than 3 years. Liver transplantation: official publication of the American Association for the Study of Liver Diseases and the International Liver Transplantation Society. 2001;7(9):811-5.

[78] Saigal S, Norris S, Muiesan P, Rela M, Heaton N, O'Grady J. Evidence of differential risk for posttransplantation malignancy based on pretransplantation cause in patients undergoing liver transplantation. Liver transplantation: official publication of the American Association

for the Study of Liver Diseases and the International Liver Transplantation Society. 2002;8(5):482-7.

[79] Bellamy CO, DiMartini AM, Ruppert K, Jain A, Dodson F, Torbenson M, et al. Liver transplantation for alcoholic cirrhosis: long term follow-up and impact of disease recurrence. *Transplantation*. 2001;72(4):619-26.

[80] Finkenstedt A, Graziadei IW, Oberaigner W, Hilbe W, Nachbaur K, Mark W, et al. Extensive surveillance promotes early diagnosis and improved survival of de novo malignancies in liver transplant recipients. American journal of transplantation: official journal of the American Society of Transplantation and the American Society of Transplant Surgeons. 2009;9(10):2355-61.

[81] Herrero JI, Alegre F, Quiroga J, Pardo F, Inarrairaegui M, Sangro B, et al. Usefulness of a program of neoplasia surveillance in liver transplantation. *A preliminary report. Clinical transplantation.* 2009;23(4):532-6.

In: Alcohol and the Liver
Editor: Gerond Lake-Bakaar
ISBN: 978-1-63484-400-0

Chapter 7

Alcoholic and Nonalcoholic Fatty Liver Disease

*Gary Trey**, *MD, MPH*
Clinical Instructor, Harvard Medical School
Attending Physician, Beth Israel Deaconess Hospital, MA, US

Abstract

Excess calorie consumption and excessive ingestion of alcohol are prevalent. Both can lead to fat accumulation in the liver and can progress to liver fibrosis, cirrhosis and hepatocellular carcinoma. When the two diseases coexist in the same individual the chances of progression are increased.

Many patients will have risk factors for both conditions and therefore may have both diseases, but these diseases are difficult to distinguish because of the similar histology. This chapter discusses each entity and addresses possible interactions in the clinical presentation.

Introduction

Ludwig and colleagues at the Mayo Clinic described in 1980 nonalcoholic steatohepatitis (NASH), which was described as histologic evidence of

* gtrey@bidmc.harvard.edu.

alcoholic hepatitis with no evidence of alcohol abuse [1]. As can be seen from the original description, alcoholic steatohepatitis (ASH) and non-alcoholic steatohepatitis are difficult to distinguish on histology. Both entities are increasing in prevalence and it is certain that many patients have both diseases. Both alcoholic liver disease (ALD) and nonalcoholic fatty liver disease (NAFLD) represent a spectrum of histology from benign fatty infiltration to cirrhosis. Ninety percent of people who drink excess alcohol will exhibit fatty filtration of the liver and about 30% of the population mainly due to obesity has nonalcoholic fatty infiltration [2].

Metabolic syndrome, which consists of BMI greater than 30, hypertension, dyslipidemia, micro-albuminuria and insulin resistance is estimated to affect 30% of the population of the United States. The syndrome is associated with obesity and NAFLD. Insulin resistance is considered to be the initiating event that causes increased hepatic triglyceride synthesis and steatosis in NAFLD. A subset will develop NASH and are at risk for cirrhosis and hepatocellular carcinoma.

Alcoholic liver disease is also increasing in prevalence affecting about 6% of the population and 20% of those will develop cirrhosis. Many patients will have risk factors for both conditions and therefore may have both diseases, but these diseases are difficult to distinguish because they have similar histology. The thrust of this chapter will be to understand each entity and the possible interactions resulting in clinical liver disease.

Fat accumulates in the liver because of decreased mitochondrial fatty acid beta-oxidation, increased fatty acid synthesis in the liver, enhanced delivery of fatty acids to the liver or deficient export of triglycerides. Every individual who consumes greater than 60 grams of alcohol daily over several years will develop fatty liver. High levels of Glycerol 3-phosphate result in increased esterification of fatty acids. Ethanol inhibits the release of VLDL from the liver. Alcohol is a mitochondrial 'poison.' Similarly, in nonalcoholic fatty liver insulin signals the liver to store fat and increase synthesis of glycogen. However, all obese patients do not accumulate excess hepatic triglycerides so it has been speculated that specific genetic factors and perhaps food choices and exercise play a role.

Hepatosteatosis refers to fat accumulation in the liver exceeding 10% by weight [3]. If hepatosteatosis occurs in the absence of 20 grams of alcohol a day in men or 10 grams in women, then the condition is felt to be nonalcoholic in etiology when drugs and other rare conditions are excluded. Examples of such drugs and conditions would include Tamoxifen, Amiodarone, Total parenteral nutrition, Bacterial overgrowth and others.

Nonalcoholic liver disease (NAFLD) is divided into: nonalcoholic fatty liver (NAFL), which is usually nonprogressive, and NASH which is usually progressive and can lead to cirrhosis and hepatocellular carcinoma The prevalence of NAFLD is 10 to 20% of the general population and 57.5 to 74% of obese individuals [4]. Ninety percent of all cases of elevated liver tests are due to NAFLD [5]. NASH is present in 12.2% of patients with type two diabetes and type two diabetes increases the risk of liver related death by 22 fold [6]. NAFLD is usually suspected in patients with elevated transaminases and is confirmed on Ultrasound or other imaging. The diagnosis of NASH at present requires a liver biopsy, but if fibrosis can be documented on transient elastography this would indicate NASH. Also degree of steatosis can be estimated by transient elastography by measuring Controlled Attenuation Parameter [7].

There are several means to distinguish between alcoholic and nonalcoholic fatty liver disease: one is look for other parts of the metabolic syndrome by measuring body mass index, insulin, glucose, A1c to look for evidence of the metabolic syndrome. Another way is to look at AST to ALT ratio. In alcoholic liver disease the AST is greater than the ALT presumably either because of alcohol induced B6 deficiency, or because of alcoholic damage to mitochondria. In B6 deficiency this change in ratio does not happen so the ratio is likely due to excess damage to mitochondria with release of mitochondrial AST. There is not much ALT in mitochondria.

In NAFLD ALT is greater than AST (liver cytosol contains greater ALT than AST). Though these ratios are not always diagnostic they can be suggestive of the cause of fatty liver disease [8]. Carbohydrate-deficient transferrin levels remain elevated for 10 days after alcohol discontinuation and thus are useful in diagnosing ASH [9].

The majority of ethanol is metabolized in the liver; it is taken up by the portal vein after being absorbed from the stomach and proximal small bowel. Acute fat accumulation in hepatocytes develops within two days of drinking greater than six drinks and can disappear within two weeks of stopping drinking alcohol. The change is usually macrovesicular with a large droplet that displaces the nucleus.

Alcohol is metabolized in the liver by alcohol dehydrogenase, cytochrome P450 2E1 and to a lesser extent catalase. The alcohol metabolites result in oxidative stress and mitochondrial damage that induce fatty accumulation. In nonalcoholic fatty liver disease fat appears to accumulate in the liver due to the effects of insulin and hyperinsulinemia, which are common in obesity and in physical deconditioning. Simple sugars, especially fructose appear to trigger fatty liver and insulin resistance. But many dietary factors play a role in development of NAFLD. Hypercaloric diets rich in saturated fat and fructose-sweetened beverages stimulate hepatic lipid accumulation. Low caloric diets, monounsaturated fats, probiotics, choline, fiber, coffee, tea and light alcohol consumption are protective against NAFLD [10]. In both entities, free fatty acids accumulate in hepatocytes and this process can be benign and not lead to further damage in a majority of people. In both entities something else happens that starts the process of inflammation and fibrosis that results in cirrhosis or alcoholic hepatitis. The debate as to what this second hit is in both these diseases is ongoing, but is felt to be due to specific genetics, virus exposure, nutritional and others.

Inflammation response in the liver is what changes steatosis to steatohepatitis in both NASH and ASH. Alcohol damages hepatocytes causing hypoxia and apoptosis. It also increases intestinal permeability to microbes and the presence of these microbes in circulation leads to inflammation as the immune system reacts to foreign antigens.

In NASH, a popular hypothesis is that inflammation results from gut bacterial translocation, which activates the immune system [11]. Overgrowth of intestinal bacteria and increased intestinal permeability are associated with NASH [12, 13]. In both disorders hepatic immune cells are exposed to components of gut microbial products, which trigger further liver injury.

The development of liver disease varies among people who drink the same amount of alcohol and eat the same amount of excess calories. Genetic factors are at play though they differ between both diseases. NAFLD has a genetic component, as family history of diabetes and Hispanic ethnicity are risk factors [14]. A genome association study of NAFLD showed that a variant of the human patatin-like phospholipase domain was associated with increased hepatic fat and inflammation and occurs in a higher frequency in Hispanics [15]. Similarly, genetic polymorphisms in alcohol metabolism in CYP2E1 and ADH and in cytokines TNF and IL-10 may play a role in alcoholic liver disease [16].

Excessive alcohol consumption, excessive calories and low physical activity are frequent in modern society. Therefore alcoholic and nonalcoholic liver disease coexist. They are difficult to distinguish as the histology is the same and our means of distinguishing them has been that the patient is drinking less than 20 grams daily. However, studies have shown that patients likely to have both diseases have increased liver damage [17]. An understanding of the clinical relevance of the components of the metabolic syndrome such as obesity, diabetes, hyperlipidemia in patients with alcoholic liver disease and their effect on disease progression is essential for understanding the progression of alcoholic liver disease.

An interesting study was recently published by Pais et al., in which they looked at 110 patients with alcohol-associated cirrhosis who had a liver transplant. Those with components of the metabolic syndrome had a 46% incidence of hepatocellular carcinoma (HCC) and those without metabolic syndrome had a 9% risk. A history of diabetes and/or overweight increased the risk of developing HCC by an odds ratio of 9:1. The findings of this study show that at least in terms of development of HCC, alcoholic and nonalcoholic fatty liver disease may be synergistic [18].

Metabolic syndrome results in higher rates of HCC in the nonalcoholic population and also in patients with other liver diseases such as hepatitis B and C [19, 20]. The progression to cirrhosis in alcoholic liver disease is modified by coexistent NAFLD. It has been shown that alcoholic patients with increased body mass have greater fibrosis [21].

Based on our far from complete understanding of the pathophysiology of NASH and ASH we can postulate on how current and future therapies might work. Obviously, both conditions would not exist if we could eliminate the causative agents alcohol and an unhealthy diet of excess simple sugars and saturated fats coupled with low caloric expenditure. In nonalcoholic liver disease, liver fat can be reduced by any form of exercise [22]. Perhaps we could stop the inflammation by changing the microbiota associated with both diseases either by the use of probiotics, antibiotics or specific nutrients to enhance beneficial bacteria or yeast and discourage harmful microbes. We can also decrease the inflammatory cascade, modify fatty deposition, decrease insulin levels and sensitivity and stop fibrosis. In alcoholic liver disease anti-inflammatory agents such as steroids have been found to be somewhat effective [23].

In nonalcoholic disease and alcoholic liver disease many substances can be postulated to help change the storage of fat in the liver and studies have been done evaluating medium chain triglycerides, vitamin E, metformin, statins and multiple other drugs without a clear therapeutic benefit [24].

Conclusion

Alcoholic and nonalcoholic liver diseases are both prevalent and can coexist. They can be distinguished on clinical and laboratory criteria. They often coexist and when they do the chances of progression to cirrhosis and hepatocellular carcinoma are increased.

REFERENCES

[1] Ludwig J, Viggiano TR, McGill DB, Oh BJ. Nonalcoholic steatohepatitis: Mayo Clinic experiences with a hitherto unnamed disease. *Mayo Clin. Proc.* 1980;55:434–438.

[2] Szczepaniak L.S, Nurenberg P, Leonard D et al. "Magnetic resonance spectroscopy to measure hepatic triglyceride content: prevalence of hepatic steatosis in the general population," *American Journal of Physiology.* 2005;288:E462–E468.

[3] Angulo P, "Medical progress: nonalcoholic fatty liver disease." *The New England Journal of Medicine,* 2002;346:1221–1231.

[4] Wanless I.R. and Lentz J.S., "Fatty liver hepatitis (steatohepatitis) and obesity: an autopsy study with analysis of risk factors," *Hepatology.* 1990;12:106–1110.

[5] Fraser A, Longnecker MP, Lawlor DA. Prevalence of elevated alanine aminotransferases among US adolescents and associated factors, *Gastro.* 2011;140:1814-1820.

[6] Z. M. Younossi, T. Gramlich, C. A. Matteoni, N. Boparai, and A. J. McCullough, "Nonalcoholic fatty liver disease in patients with type 2 diabetes," *Clinical Gastroenterology and Hepatology.* 2004:2: 262–265.

[7] Myers R.P., Pollett, A. Kirsch, R. Controlled Attenuation Parameter (CAP) A Noninvasive Method for the Detection of Hepatic Steatosis Based on Transient Elastography. *Liver International.* 2012;32:902-910.

[8] Sorbi D, Boynton J, Lindor KD. The ratio of aspartate aminotransferase to alanine aminotransferase: potential value in differentiating nonalcoholic steatohepatitis from alcoholic liver disease. *Am Journal Gastro.* 1999;94(4):1018-22.

[9] J.R. Delanghe, A. Helander, J.P.M. Wielders, J.M. Pekelharing, H.J. Roth, F. Schellenberg, C. Born, E. Yagmur, W. Gentzer, H. Althaus. Development and multicenter evaluation of the N latex CDT direct immunonephelometric assay for serum carbohydrate-deficient transferrin. *Clin. Chem.* 53 (2007), pp. 1116–1121.

[10] Fan JG, Cao HX. Role of diet and nutritional management in non-alcoholic fatty liver disease. *J Gastroenterol Hepatol.* 2013 Dec;28 Suppl 4:81-7. doi: 10.1111/jgh.12244.

[11] Szabo G., Iracheta-Vellve. Inflammasome activation in the Liver: Focus on alcoholic and non-alcoholic steatohepatitis. *Clin Res Hepatol and Gastro.* 2015;39:S18-S23.

[12] Miele L, Valenza V, La Torre G, Montalto M, Cammarota G, Ricci R, et al. Increased intestinal permeability and tight junction alterations in nonalcoholic fatty liver disease, *Hepatology.* 2009;49:1877–87.

[13] Mouzaki M, Comelli E, Arendt B et al. Intestinal Microbiota in Patients with Nonalcoholic Fatty Liver Disease. *Hepatology.* 2013;58:120-127.

[14] loomba R, Abraham M., Unalp A, et al. Nonalcoholic Steatohepatitis Clinical Research network. Association between diabetes, family history of diabetes, and risk of nonalcoholic steatohepatitis and fibrosis. *Hepatology.* 2012;56:829-834.

[15] Pirazzi C, Adiels M, Burza MA, et al. Patatin-like phospholipase domain-containing 3 (PNLAS) 1148M (rs738409) affects hepatic VLDL secretion in humans and in vitro. *J Hepatol.* 2012;57:1276-1282.

[16] Shukla SD, Velazquez J, French SW, et al. Emerging role of epigenetics in the actions of alcohol. *Alcohol Clin Exp Res.* 2008;32:1525-34.

[17] Naveau S. Giraud V, Borotto E, et al. Excess weight is a risk factor for alcoholic liver disease. *Hepatology* 1997;25:108-111.

[18] Pais R. Lebray P, Rousseau G, et al. Nonalcoholic Fatty liver Disease Increases the Risk of Hepatocellular Carcinoma in Patients With Alcohol-associated Cirrhosis Awaiting liver Transplants. *Clinical Gastro and Hepatology* 2015;13:992-999.

[19] Welzel Tm, Graubard Bl, Zeuzem S, et al. Metabolic syndrome increases the risk of primary liver cancer in the United States: a study in the SEER-Medicare database. *Hepatology* 2011;54: 463-471.

[20] Chen CL, Yang HI, Yang WS, et al. Metabolic factors and risk of hepatocellular carcinoma by chronic hepatitis B/C infection: a follow-up study in Taiwan. *Gastroenterology* 2008;135:111-112.

[21] Raynard B, Balian A, Falik D, et al. Risk Factors of fibrosis in alcohol-induced liver disease. *Hepatology* 2002;35:635-638.

[22] Keating SE, Hackett DA, Parker HM et al. Effect of aerobic exercise training dose on liver fat and visceral adiposity. *Journal of Hepatology* 2015;63:174-182.

[23] Thursz MR, Richardson P, Allison M, et al. Prednisone or pentoxifylline for alcoholic hepatitis. *N Engl J Med* 2015;372:1619-1628.

[24] Pearlman M, Loomba R. State of the treatment of nonalcoholic steatohepatitis. *Curr Opin Gastro* 2014;30:223-237.

In: Alcohol and the Liver
Editor: Gerond Lake-Bakaar
ISBN: 978-1-63484-400-0

Chapter 8

PATHOLOGIC FEATURES AND MECHANISMS IN ALCOHOLIC LIVER DISEASE

Imad A. Nasser[1,*], *MD*
[1]Department of Pathology, Beth Israel Deaconess Medical Center, Boston, MA, US

ABSTRACT

Chronic alcohol abuse is a cause of significant mobidity and mortality in the US and other countries. The liver is one of the major organs affected. This chapter addresses the pathological changes in alcoholic liver disease.

Alcohol induced liver injury progresses from simple steatosis to steatohepatitis with perisinusoidal fibrosis and finally to cirrhosis. About 20%-30% of patients with steatosis develop alcoholic hepatitis and 16% of patients with steatohepatitis progress to cirrhosis.

We discuss specific forms of presentation of alcoholic liver disease. As an example, foamy degeneration is a rare lesion characterized by hepatocytes filled with small fat droplets with increase in size of the cells.

Potential mechanisms of alcohol induced liver injury are also discussed.

* E-mail: inasser@bidmc.harvard.edu.

Alcohol consumption can cause major health issues in certain individuals. One of the major organs that can be affected is the liver. Depending on multiple factors, including the amount and duration of intake, hepatic injury can range in severity from steatosis to the development of cirrhosis and hepatocellular carcinoma. About 90% of ingested alcohol is absorbed in the upper GI tract (stomach and small bowel, particularly the jejunum) and diffusely distributed throughout the body [1]. Approximately 90% of ingested alcohol is metabolized in the liver [2].

Alcohol induced injury starts as simple steatosis and with continued exposure, progresses to steatohepatitis with the development of perisinusoidal fibrosis and finally cirrhosis. In steatohepatitis, Mallory bodies, ballooning degeneration, mega-mitochondria, and occlusive lesions of terminal hepatic venules can be seen [3]. Alcoholic hepatitis is a necroinflammatory process that can progress to cirrhosis.

Steatosis occurs as a result of metabolism of ethanol in the liver. Alcohol is absorbed in the stomach and small bowel, and the metabolism starts in the gastrointestinal tract, where alcohol dehydrogenase is present [4]. It converts alcohol into acetaldehyde, however, this contributes little to the overall metabolism, which occurs mainly on the liver. In the liver, in addition to the alcohol dehydrogenase pathway in the cytosol, under chronic and heavy alcohol intake conditions the microsomal ethanol oxidation system present in the smooth endoplasmic reticulum which acts through the cytochrome P450 family, plays significant role; catalase present in the peroxisomes plays a minor role. At high concentration of ethanol, the cytochrome P450 enzymes (CYP2E1, 1A2, and 3A4), which are present mainly in microsomes, convert ethanol into acetaldehyde and are present at increased levels. The cytochrome P450 family, particularly CYP2E, are mainly expressed in the centrivenular zone 3 hepatocytes of the liver. This is why the earliest change, steatosis, is first seen in this zone (Figure 1).

Alcohol dehydrogenase is present in the cytosol where it converts alcohol to acetaldehyde and other metabolites. Acetaldehyde is then converted to acetate by acetaldehyde dehydrogenase. Acetaldehyde is the key toxin in alcohol-induced liver injury, causing cellular damage and inflammation. In this reaction nicotinamide adenine dinucleotide (NAD+) is reduced by two electrons to NADH generating a highly reduced environment in hepatocytes.

Acetate can be incorporated into acetyl-CoA, a mitochondrial fuel, for use in Krebs cycle oxidation and fatty acid synthesis. This conversion is catalyzed by the acyl-CoA synthetase and contributes to lipid synthesis and energy generation.

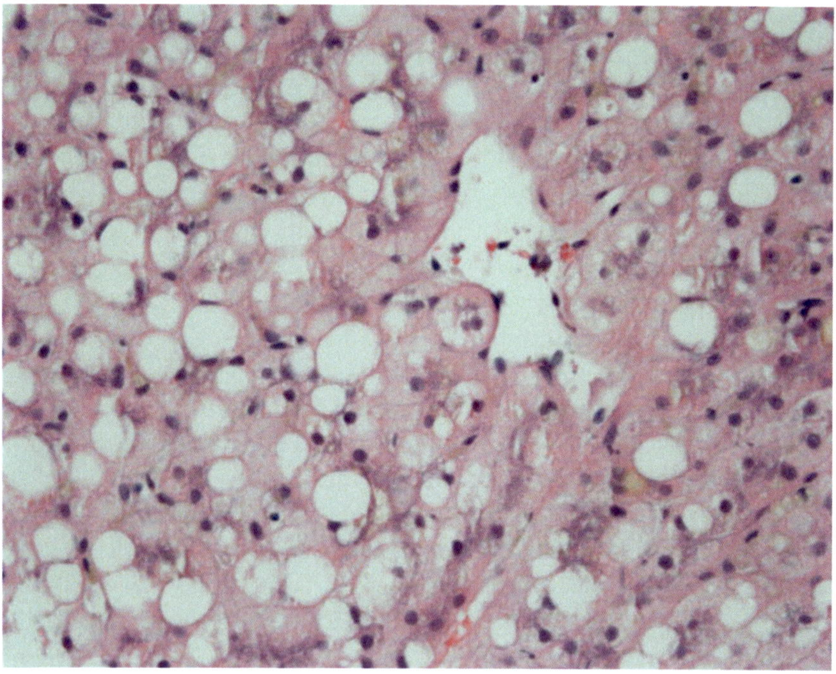

Figure 1. Steatosis in centrivenular (zone 3) region. Macrovesicular steatosis with a large clear intracytoplasmic vacuole that displaces the nuclei to periphery in individual hepatocytes (H&E stain).

Excess NADH and the increased NADH/NAD ratio may promote conversion of acetate molecules are into fat, which are then esterified with glycerol to form triglycerides. Cytosolic lipid droplets are formed and give the microscopic appearance of hepatic steatosis. They start as microvesiscles or small droplets (1 to 2 micrometers in diameter) and later coalesce or enlarge to form macrovesicles or large droplets (Figure 1).

In general, the morphologic features of microvesicular steatosis are multiple fat globules present within the cytoplasm that do not displace the hepatocyte nucleus, while in macrovesicular steatosis the fat globule is singular, large and displaces the nucleus to periphery and compresses it.

Acetaldehyde is a highly reactive and toxic byproduct that forms within hepatocytes that may contribute to tissue damage. It forms a variety of protein and DNA adducts that promote glutathione depletion, lipid peroxidation, and mitochondrial damage. The acetaldehyde produced from alcohol oxidation is rapidly metabolized into NADH and acetate by aldehyde dehydrogenase (ALDH) in mitochondria. In addition, alcohol exposure impairs delivery of

VLDL-containing vesicles from the Golgi apparatus to the hepatocyte cell membrane for release into the circulation [5], so lipoprotein lipids accumulate in the Golgi apparatus.

There are genes encoding for alcohol-dehydrogenase (ADH), aldehyde-dehydrogenase (ALDH) and C2-promoter allele of the gene coding for cytochrome CYP2E1. Gene polymorphism studies by Chao et al. suggest that genes encoding for enzymes that metabolize both ethanol and acetaldehyde can change the predisposition to alcohol dependence, sensitivity to alcohol and degree of hepatic injury induced by alcohol consumption [6].

Another form of steatosis in alcoholic liver disease is alcoholic foamy degeneration described by Uchida et al. [7]. This injury is characterized by enlarged hepatocytes filled with small fat droplets within the cytoplasm that have centrally placed nuclei [8]. This is a rare lesion and is reported in 0.8% and 2.3% in two series of alcoholic liver disease.

Ballooning of hepatocytes is another morphologic feautre that can be seen with alcoholic liver damage. Hepatocyte ballooning (Figure 2) leads to cell lysis and death. Hepatocellular ballooning occurs due to cytoplasmic accumulation of lipids, fluid and protein. The cell becomes swollen and enlarged with a centrally placed nucleus and cytoplasmic stringing. Hepatocyte ballooning is the result of severe cell injury involving depletion of adenosine triphosphate (ATP) and an increase in intracellular Ca^{2+}. Oxidative damage that occurs during alcohol metabolism disrupts cytoplasmic and nuclear proteins, organelle membranes and proteins, and DNA. Mitochondrial oxygen reduction becomes impaired leading to mitochondrial dysfunction which is characterized by permeability of both the outer and inner mitochondrial membranes. Loss of the inner mitochondrial membrane barrier leads to collapse of ion gradients and decreased oxidative phosphorylation. This leads to ATP depletion and destruction of the cytoskeleton. Ballooning degeneration ends in necrosis, whereby the cell undergoes karyolysis and release of cellular constituents into the extracellular environment.

Another histological feature that can be seen in ballooned hepatocytes are Mallory bodies or alcoholic hyaline described by Frank Burr Mallory in 1911 [9]. Mallory bodies are intracytoplasmic eosinophilic, homogeneous, rope-like material that may be short and irregular or long and can form a complete or open ring around the nucleus (Figure 2).

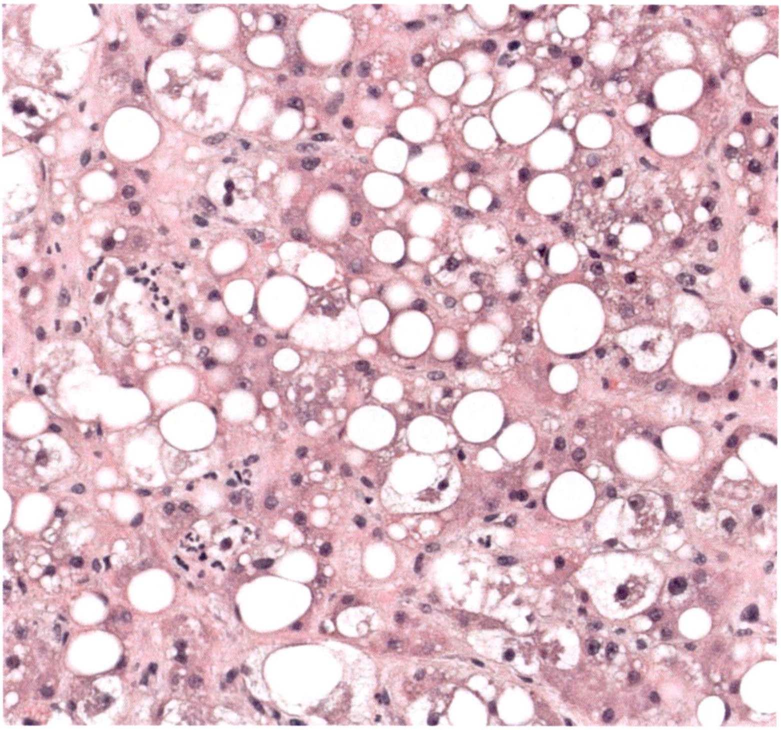

Figure 2. Hepatocytes with ballooning degeneration. Malloy's bodies with surrounding neutophils are seen at 11:00 o'clock. H&E stain.

Mallory bodies may be comprised of various proteins including CK8 and CK18, which comprise the intermediate filaments present within the cytoskeleton of hepatocytes.. In addition, Mallory bodies may have ubiquitin binding protein p62, heat-shock proteins (HSPs) 70 and 25. These cytokeratin bundles may bind to TNF receptor 2 (TNFR2), thus leading to TNF-α–induced activation which induces aggregation of neutrophils (Figure 2). Three types of Mallory bodies have been identified by electron microscopy. [10]. Type I consists of bundles of filaments (5-20 nm thick) in parallel arrays; type II is composed of randomly oriented fibrils and type III consists of a granular or amorphous, markedly electron-dense substance containing only scattered fibrils.

About 20%-30% of patients with steatosis develop alcoholic hepatitis and 16% of patients with steatohepatitis will develop cirrhosis [11].

Short and long term ethanol consumption can disrupt the epithelial barrier of the GI tract which results in increased intestinal permeability and enhanced movement of luminal antigens such as bacteria and endotoxins into the portal circulation. This can lead to Kupffer cell activation in the liver and cytokine release, which may consequently result in liver injury [12].

Cytokines secreted by activated Kupffer cells and other inflammatory cells stimulate the stellate cells to divide and secrete large amounts of extracellular matrix. This usually occurs in areas of hepatocellular necrosis and inflammation. The perisinusoidal space of Disse usually contains delicate interspersed strands of fibrillar collagen types III and IV. When the stellate cells are activated, they deposit a dense matrix of basement membrane–type material. Extracellular matrix proteins normally present in basement membranes are deposited within the space of Disse, creating a barrier for exchange between hepatocytes and sinusoidal blood. This appears as perisinusoidal fibrosis on microscopic examination by trichrome stain (Figure 3). In addition, portal tract fibrogenesis develops later and concomitantly with perisinusoidal fibrosis.

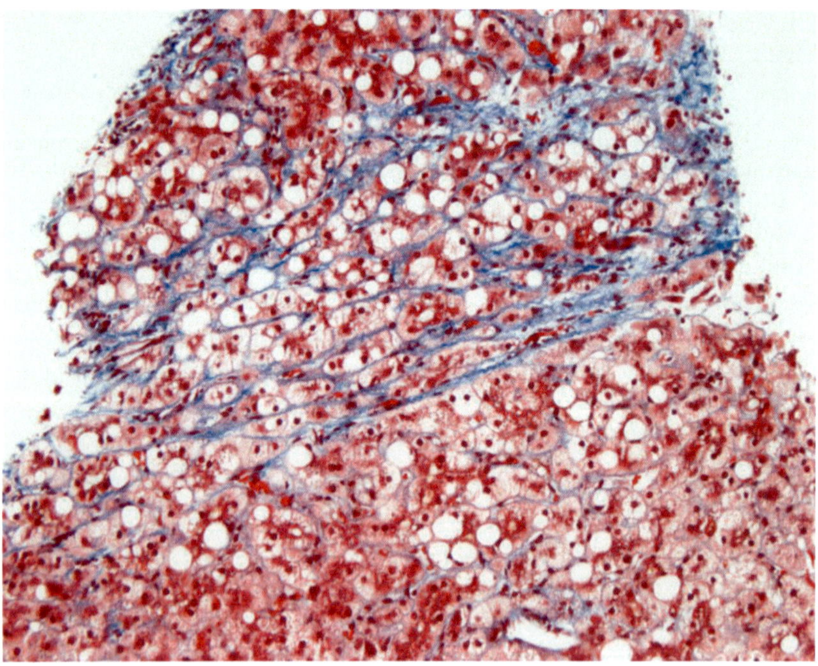

Figure 3. Tichrome stain demonstrate typical perisinusoidal fibrosis.

Cells that can contribute to portal and septal fibrosis include fibroblasts that surround bile ducts and those at the interface between the portal tracts and hepatocytes as well as myofibroblasts present around the portal vein and hepatic artery. The end stage is the development of cirrhosis which starts as micronodules and later and mixed macro-nodular and micro-nodular cirrhosis.

Another histologic feature seen in steatohepatitis is canalicular cholestasis. If present, it is usually minimal (Figure 4). In addition, the toxic damage results in abnormal mitochondria some of which are large and can be seen on H&E and are called megamitochondria. Most often they are round, eosinophilic and located in zone 3. Megamitochondria can have irregular shapes and contain paracrystalline and granular inclusions and can sometimes be small.

After cessation of alcohol, the first histologic change is the disappearance of steatosis. It can take from a few days up to in 3-4 weeks to completely disappear, depending on the extent. Mallory bodies are said to disappear in 6 to 12 weeks in humans [13], but can take up to six months.

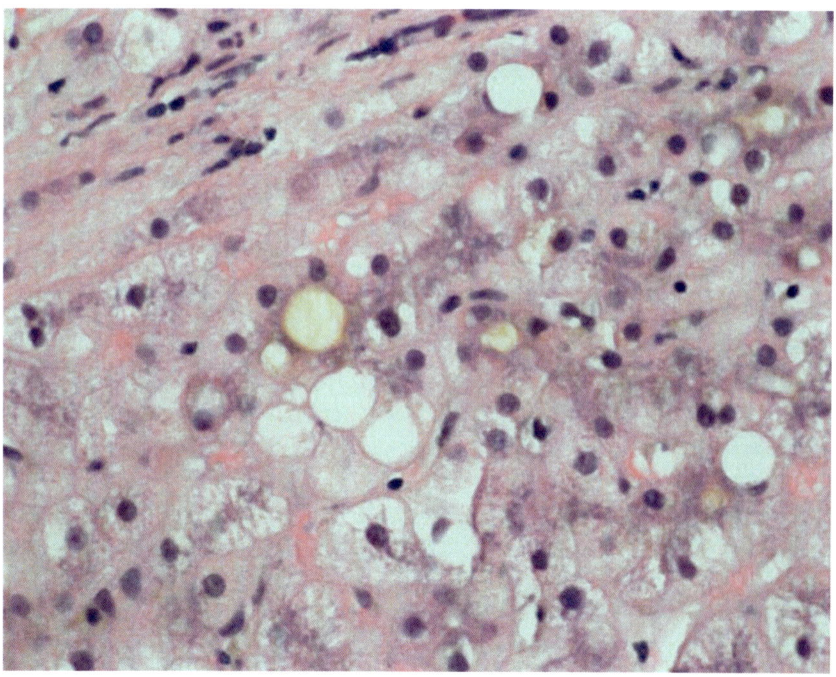

Figure 4. Canalicular cholestasis in alcoholic hepatitis.

The 3 forms of alcoholic liver disease

Feature	Fatty Liver Disease	Alcoholic Hepatitis	Cirrhosis
Steatosis	•••	••	••• to •[a]
Hepatocyte ballooning	—	•••	•
Mallory bodies	—	••	•
Inflammation	—	•••	•
Hepatocyte necrosis	—	•••	••
Regeneration	—	•	••
Fibrosis	—	••	••••

The relative proportions of 7 morphologic findings are given as the number of dots.
[a] The degree of steatosis in alcoholic cirrhosis depends on whether the cirrhosis developed in the absence (•••) or presence (••) of alcoholic hepatitis. Regardless, with the passage of time steatosis in the cirrhotic liver may diminish to a minimal value (•).

Figure 5. Forms of alcoholic liver disease with histological features as illustrated by Crawford [14].

A summary of common histologic features in alcoholic liver disease is shown in this table (Figure 5) by Crawford [14].

References

[1] Levitt M. D., Li R., DeMaster E. G., Elson M., Furne J., Levitt D. G. Am J. Physiol. Use of measurements of ethanol absorption from stomach and intestine to assess human ethanol metabolism. *Am. J. Physiol.,* 1997; 273(4 Pt 1):G951-7.

[2] Schuckit M. A. Alcohol and alcoholism. In: Kasper D. L., Braunwald E., Fauci A. S., Hauser S. L., Longo D. L., Jameson J. L., editors. Harrison's Principles of internal medicine. NewYork: McGraw-Hill Medical Publishing Division. 2005:2562-2566.

[3] Ishak K. G., Zimmerman H. J., Ray M. B. Alcoholic Liver Disease: Pathologic, Pathogenetic and Clinical Aspects. *Alcoholismcil Inical And Experimental Research,* 1991;15(1): pages 45–66.

[4] Cederbaum, A. I. Alcohol metabolism. *Clin. Liver. Dis.*, 2012;16, 667–685.

[5] R. F. Peters T. J., Cairns S. R. Analysis and subcellular localization of lipid in alcoholic liver disease. *Alcohol,* 1985;2:447–51.

[6] Chao Y. C., Liou S. R., Chung Y. Y., et al. Polymorphism of alcohol and aldehydedehydrogenase genes and alcoholic cirrhosis in Chinese patients. *Hepatology,* 1994;19: 360–6.

[7] Uchida T., Kao H., Quispe-Sjogren M., Peters R. L. Alcoholic foamy degeneration--a pattern of acute alcoholic injury of the liver. *Gastroenterology,* 1983; 84(4):683-92.

[8] MacSween R. N. M., Burt A. D. Histologic spectrum of alcoholic liver disease. *Semin. Liver Dis.,* 1986; 6:221-232.

[9] Mallory, F. B. Bulletin of the Johns Hopkins Hospital. 1911. Cirrhosis of the liver; p. 22.

[10] Yokoo H., Minick O. T., Batti F., Kent G.: Morphologic variants of alcoholic hyalin. *Am. J. Pathol.,* 1972;69:25-40.

[11] Pateria P., de Boer B., MacQuillan G. Liver abnormalities in drug and substance abusers. *Best Pract. Res. Clin. Gastroenterol.,* 2013; 27:577-596.

[12] Adachi Y., Bradford B. U., Gao W., Bojes H. K., Thurman R. G. Inactivation of Kupffer cells prevents early alcohol-induced liver injury. *Hepatology,* 1994; 20: 453-460.

[13] Tsutsumi M., Lasker J. M., Shimizu M., Rosman A. S., Lieber C. S. The intralobular distribution of ethanol-inducible P450II EI in rat and human liver. 1989. *Hepatology,* 10:437-446.

[14] Crawford J. M. Histologic Findings in Alcoholic Liver Disease. *Clin. Liver Dis.,* 2012;16 699–716.

In: Alcohol and the Liver
Editor: Gerond Lake-Bakaar
ISBN: 978-1-63484-400-0

Chapter 9

ALCOHOL AND THE LIVER: ROLE OF MITOCHONDRIA

Alfredo Saavedra-Molina[1], Héctor Riveros-Rosas[2], Adriana Julián-Sánchez[2], Rocío Montoya-Pérez[1] and Ruth Noriega-Cisneros[1]

[1]Instituto de Investigaciones Químico-Biológicas,
Universidad Michoacana de San Nicolás de Hidalgo,
Morelia, Mich. México

[2]Departamento de Bioquímica, Facultad de Medicina, UNAM, México

ABSTRACT

Alcohol consumption, abuse, and dependence are social problems that emerged as a consequence of industrialization. Ethanol itself is a toxic metabolite that produces deleterious effects like fatty liver despite adequate diets. It is evident that the net effect of alcohol consumption on health is detrimental and is a causal factor in 60 types of diseases and injuries, and a component that causes in 200 others. The liver is the main site of ethanol oxidation, and is extremely vulnerable to alcoholic damage. The most prevalent types of alcoholic liver diseases are fatty liver, alcoholic hepatitis, and cirrhosis. Heavy drinkers and alcoholics may progress from fatty liver to alcoholic hepatitis to cirrhosis, and it is estimated that 10 percent to 15 percent of alcoholics will develop cirrhosis. A number of mechanisms have been postulated for the pathogenesis of alcoholic injuries and diseases, including toxicity of ethanol and its metabolite acetaldehyde, the primary metabolic product of ethanol. In addition, oxidative stress, and accumulation of fatty acid ethyl esters also contribute to alcohol-associated complications. Interestingly, in all these mechanisms of toxicity, mitochondria play a central role. Oxidative pathways are by far the main pathways responsible of ethanol clearance. Currently, in animals there are three non homologous $NAD(P)^+$-dependent alcohol dehydrogenases (ADH) protein families that possess different structures and mechanisms of reaction. The Microsomal Ethanol Oxidizing System (MEOS) system catalyzes the oxidation from ethanol to acetaldehyde, coupling this reaction to the oxidation of an NADPH molecule, and the reduction of an oxygen molecule to form hydrogen peroxide. Mitochondria participate with the conversion of acetaldehyde into acetate and the generation of increased amounts of NADH. Mitochondria play an important role in the alcohol metabolism via the enzyme ALDH; this enzyme catalyzes the oxidation of acetaldehyde into acetate. The acetaldehyde is capable of escape into the blood stream and leads to damage to biomolecules such as lipids, proteins and nucleic acids, which results in the toxic side effects that are associated with alcohol consumption. Mitochondrial dysfunction results in decreased ATP synthesis and increased reactive oxygen species (ROS) production, which can compromise the survival, function and regeneration capacity of hepatocytes, especially in pathological conditions such as cirrhosis, in which chronic damage in liver causes changes in mitochondria. In cells, the mitochondrial electron transport chain (ETC) is one of the most important sources of ROS. Ethanol metabolism executes conditions that promote ROS formation by mitochondria, effects that may be enhanced by a decrease in the mitochondrial antioxidant systems. Either acute or chronic ethanol consumption produces excessive ROS, mitochondrial dysfunction and endoplasmic reticulum stress in liver. It is clear that antioxidants may play a role in the treatment of alcoholic liver disease. Plants and plant derived compounds have been shown to to improve symptoms. However clinical benefit is still far from proven.

1. Introduction

One hundred years ago Federico Battelli and Lina Stern (1909) found that extracts from various animal tissues are able to oxidize alcohol, and they made the first preparation of a soluble alcohol dehydrogenase from horse liver. Because the manufacture and consumption of alcoholic beverages are ancient practices common to nearly all cultures, and their origins are associated in most cases, to the occurrence of agriculture (Phillips, 2014), it was considered that this capability is inherent to animal metabolism and no one questioned the presence of an alcohol dehydrogenase (ADH) in animals. Indeed, ADH activity is widely distributed in all kinds of animals (Hernández-Tobías et al., 2011). However, it is important to point out that alcohol consumption abuse as a social problem emerged as a consequence of industrialization, when availability of large quantities of cheap and stronger alcoholic beverages was possible (Nikelly, 1994; Anderson and Baumberg, 2006). Unsurprisingly, this lead to sharp increases in the consumption of alcohol (Knapp, 1998). Before the technological developments from the XVII through XIX Centuries, the manufacture of fermented beverages was mainly a family business, comprising a relatively scarce and expensive commodity. Therefore, in pre-industrial societies, drinking were allowed only in cultural prescribed occasions, as part of traditional, organized activities in which large segments of the community participates (Nikelly, 1994). On these conditions, the pathological consequences of alcohol abuse were infrequent (Singer, 1986). The manufacture of distilled beverages (spirits) date from XIII century, but were almost solely used as medicines for several hundred years, and commonly called as *aqua vitae* or "water of life", and were removed from the doctor's cabinet until XX century (Anderson and Baumberg, 2006). Indeed, until the first half of XX Century was considered that the toxic effects observed in alcoholics were due to concomitant malnutrition and not to ethanol (or its metabolites) *per se*, (e.g., Best et al., 1949). The pioneering studies performed by Charles S. Lieber and coworkers proved, for first time, that ethanol itself is a toxic metabolite that produce deleterious effects like fatty liver despite adequate diets (Lieber et al., 1965).

Today, it is evident that the net effect of alcohol consumption on health is detrimental (Herd, 1992), and is a causal factor in 60 types of diseases and injuries, and a component cause in 200 others (WHO, 2011). Overall, alcohol abuse is responsible for 3 - 8% of all global deaths (Rehm et al., 2009), and 4% of the global burden of disease is attributable to alcohol, which accounts for about as much death and disability globally as tobacco and hypertension (Room et al., 2005). Indeed, the economic costs associated with the abuse of alcohol amount to more than 1% of the gross national product in high-income and middle-income countries (Rehm et al., 2009). Interestingly, total public spending for hospital-based treatment of alcohol abuse exceed, 3 times on average, that for illegal drug treatment in Europe (Lievens et al., 2014).

Worldwide, alcohol consumption average is 6.1 L of pure alcohol (defined as 100% ethanol) per adult per year (WHO, 2011), although there are wide variations. The highest consumption levels can be found in the developed world. Even if most of the adult population drinks at low-risk levels most of the time or abstains altogether, the broad range of alcohol consumption patterns, from daily heavy drinking to occasional hazardous drinking, creates significant public health and safety problems in nearly all countries (WHO, 2011).

The liver is the main site of ethanol oxidation, and is extremely vulnerable to alcoholic damage (Guo and Ren, 2010). The most prevalent types of alcoholic liver disease are fatty liver, alcoholic hepatitis, and cirrhosis (Mann et al., 2003). A conclusive demonstration of liver damage due to ethanol was presented by Lelbach (1974), who concluded that the risk of developing cirrhosis is a function of both quantity and duration of alcohol consumption. Heavy drinkers and alcoholics may progress from fatty liver to alcoholic hepatitis to cirrhosis, and it is estimated that 10 percent to 15 percent of alcoholics will develop cirrhosis (Mann et al., 2003).

A number of mechanisms have been postulated for the pathogenesis of alcoholic injuries and diseases, including toxicity of ethanol and its metabolite acetaldehyde, the primary metabolic product of ethanol (e.g., Mello et al., 2008). In addition, oxidative stress (Albano, 2008), and accumulation of fatty acid ethyl esters (Laposata and Lange, 1986) also contribute to alcohol-associated complications. Interestingly, in all these mechanisms of toxicity, mitochondria play a central role as will be exposed in the following sections.

2. Ethanol Metabolism

Ethanol Absorption

In humans, diet is the main source of alcohol. Once ethanol is ingested, it begins to be absorbed immediately through the mucous epithelium of the mouth and as vapour in the lungs (Batt, 1989); however, the amount of ethanol that is absorbed through these two pathways is negligible. Thus, it can be considered that all the ingested alcohol goes to the stomach, where it is absorbed by simple diffusion through the epithelium of the stomach and small intestine (Watson, 1989); only small quantities of alcohol reach the colon. Ethanol is absorbed from the GI tract by simple diffusion in a way entirely similar to that of water, due to its small molecular size, moderate lipid solubility, and excellent water solubility (Crabb et al., 1987). Thus, once ethanol arrives at the stomach it is absorbed in small proportion toward the bloodstream through the gastric mucosae (approximately 20 – 30%) while the largest amount is channeled through the same gastric emptying toward the small intestine (Batt, 1989; Elamin et al., 2013). It is in the small intestine (principally duodenum and jejunum) where the major part of absorption of ethanol is performed. The rate of alcohol absorption depends mainly on the rate of gastric emptying and the concentration of alcohol, and is more rapid in the fasted state (Riveros-Rosas et al., 1997). Thus, the blood alcohol concentration is determined by the amount of alcohol consumed, the presence or absence of food, and the rate of alcohol metabolism (Cederbaum, 2012). A small proportion of ethanol is excreted unchanged: 1–5% via the lungs, 0.1–0.5% in sweat, and 0.5–2% in urine (Holford, 1987).

Fate of Ethanol in the Body

Once ethanol is in blood, it is distributed over all the bodily fluids, crossing freely through all of the biological membranes (Watson, 1989). Thus, the equilibrium concentration of alcohol in a tissue depends on the relative water content of that tissue (Cederbaum, 2012). Therefore, in the terminal ileum and colon, ethanol concentrations approximate those in blood (Elamin et al., 2013). Women, who have a smaller proportion of bodily fluids than men (53% vs. 61.8%), reach the highest levels of ethanol in blood even if both men and women ingest equivalent amounts of alcohol (Watson, 1989; Batt, 1989). Indeed, ethanol is not distributed in body fat (Batt, 1989).

Ethanol Metabolism in the Liver

Ethyl alcohol absorbed from the gastrointestinal tract is rapidly channeled toward the portal vein and from there, carried directly to the liver to be metabolized. On mammals, ethanol can be metabolized through several oxidative and non-oxidative enzymatic systems (Riveros-Rosas et al., 1997), illustrated in Figure 1. Oxidative pathways are by far the main pathways responsible of ethanol clearance. Thus, ethanol is oxidized to acetaldehyde, which is further oxidized to acetate, the same final metabolite produced from the main macronutrients (carbohydrates, fats, and proteins). Approximately 90% of ingested ethanol is oxidized in the body, principally in the liver (extra hepatic metabolism of ethanol is small) (Lieber, 2005). This relative organ specificity, coupled with the high energy content of ethanol (7 kcal/g and the lack of effective feedback control of its oxidation rate in the liver, may result in a displacement, by ethanol, up to 90% of the liver's normal metabolic substrates, and probably explains why ethanol disposal produces striking metabolic imbalances in the liver (Lieber, 2005). The extent to which ethanol becomes the preferred fuel for the total body has been demonstrated: it decreased total body fat oxidation by 79% and protein oxidation by 39%, and almost completely abolished the 249% rise in carbohydrate oxidation seen after glucose infusion (Shelmet et al., 1988).

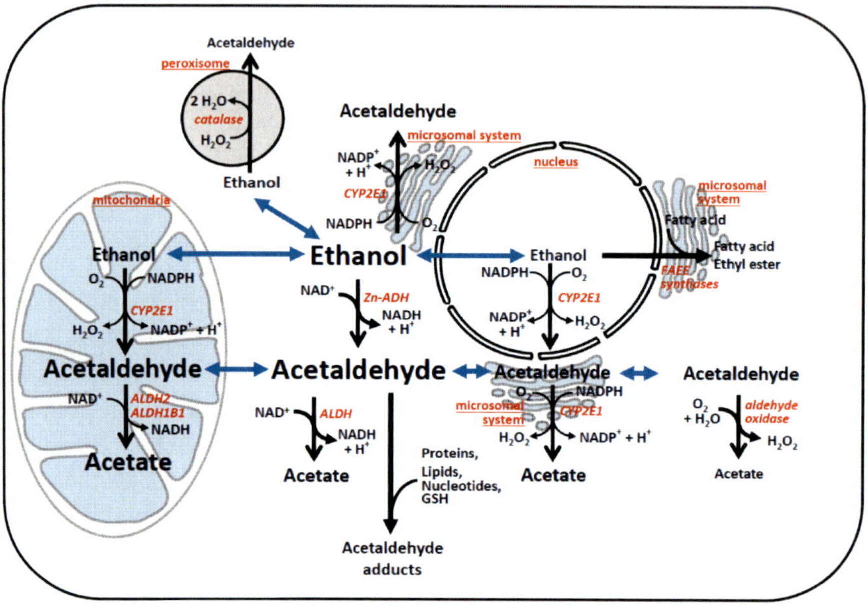

Figure 1. Enzymes involved in hepatic ethanol metabolism are distributed among different cellular compartments. Enzymes are indicated in red italics, black arrows indicate metabolic reactions and blue arrows metabolite movement through different cell compartments (ethanol and acetaldehyde can cross freely all biological membranes). The font size used to indicate the different metabolites is proportional to the relative flux through the illustrated metabolic reactions.

Alcohol Dehydrogenases (ADHs)

Currently, in animals there are three non homologous $NAD(P)^+$-dependent ADH protein families that possess different structures and mechanisms of reaction (Hernández-Tobías et al., 2011). Type I ADHs are zinc-containing enzymes (Zn-ADHs) with approximately 350 residues per subunit, and they belong to the "medium-chain" dehydrogenase/reductase superfamily (Riveros-Rosas et al., 2003). Type II ADHs lack metal cofactor, contain circa 250 residues per subunit, and belong to the "short-chain" dehydrogenase/reductase superfamily (Ladenstein et al., 2008). The most studied ADH inside this group is the short-chain ADH from the fruit fly *Drosophila melanogaster*, and therefore is described also as the "insect" ADH; indeed, the distribution of these enzymes is limited to insects of the order diptera (Hernández-Tobías et al., 2011). Type III ADHs are described as "iron-dependent/activated" enzymes, contain nearly 385 residues per subunit, and belong to the iron-containing alcohol dehydrogenase (Fe-ADH) superfamily (Reid and Fewson, 1994). However, in vertebrates, including humans, contribution of type II and type III ADHs on ethanol oxidation rate is negligible; therefore, Zn-ADHs can be considered as the only ADH type that contributes to ethanol metabolism on vertebrates (Hernández-Tobías et al., 2011). Indeed, flux control analysis show that Zn-ADHs are the major enzymes modulating ethanol oxidation rate (Yao et al., 2010).

Humans possess seven *Zn-Adh* genes originated by tandem gene duplication, which are located on the same gene cluster at chromosome 4q22–23 (González-Duarte and Albalat, 2005). Zn-ADHs have broad substrate specificity, and surprisingly, this enzymes display a higher catalytic efficiency for many endogenous substrates in comparison with ethanol (Riveros-Rosas et al., 1997). The maximum reported efficiencies of Zn-ADH isozymes from mammals, with ethanol are 300 mM^{-1} min^{-1} (Han et al., 1998). This value of catalytic efficiency is low in comparison with endogenous substrates like dopamine metabolites (190,000 mM^{-1} min^{-1}) (Mardh and Vallee, 1986), S-nitrosoglutathione (110,000 mM^{-1} min^{-1}) (Staab et al., 2008), 4-hydroxynonenal (28,000 mM^{-1} min^{-1}) (Sellin et al., 1991), serotonin metabolites (12,000 mM^{-1} min^{-1}) (Svensson et al., 1999), all-*trans*-retinol (4,500 mM^{-1} min^{-1}) (Han et al., 1998), 20-hydroxy-leukotriene B_4 (983 mM^{-1} min^{-1}) (Gotoh et al., 1990), or steroid metabolites (400 mM^{-1} min^{-1}) (McEvily et al., 1988). However, because the concentration of endogenous substrates in the body are in the micromolar range, and ethanol concentrations in alcoholics or even social drinkers are in the millimolar range, ingestion of alcoholic beverages might impair severely the metabolism of the above mentioned endogenous substrates, because ethanol can function as a competitive inhibitor (Riveros-Rosas et al., 1997). On other hand, Lieber and DeCarli have reported hepatic ADH activity as not inducible by ethanol in primates as well as most other animal species (Lieber, 2005). Thus, oxidation of ethanol via Zn-ADH can explain various metabolic effects of ethanol but does not account for the development of alcohol-tolerance (Lieber, 2004). This support the hypothesis that enzymogenesis of Zn-dependent ADHs is not triggered by ethanol, and suggest that the participation of Zn-ADHs on ethanol metabolism can be considered as incidental, and not adaptive (Hernández-Tobías et al., 2011).

Microsomal Ethanol Oxidizing System (MEOS)

This system was studied for the first time by Lieber et al. at the end of the 60s (Lieber and DeCarli, 1968; Rubin et al., 1968) from an initial report by Orme-Johnson and Ziegler (1965), where they described parallel increments in the capacity to metabolize drugs and ethanol, with total activity of cytochrome P450 in the smooth endoplasmic reticulum of hepatic cells. In this way, from these initial reports, the existence of a new pathway for ethanol oxidation, dependent on cytochrome P-450, was quickly described. The MEOS system catalyzes the oxidation from ethanol to acetaldehyde, coupling this reaction to oxidation of an NADPH molecule, and the reduction of an oxygen molecule to form hydrogen peroxide.

Cytochrome P450s are a superfamily of heme enzymes that comprise 57 genes in humans, which are involved in the oxidation of steroids, fatty acids, eicosanoids, retinoids, etc., as well as in the elimination of numerous xenobiotics ingested from the environment (Nebert et al., 2013). Different types of cytochrome P450 are capable of catalyzing the ethanol oxidation, although the most efficient is cytochrome P450 2E1, also called CYP2E1, or simply 2E1 (Nelson et al., 1993). Highest levels of cytochromes P450 are found in the liver, where they are present mainly in the endoplasmic reticulum or microsomal fraction (Cederbaum, 2012), but also has been reported in other subcellular locations including mitochondria (Anandatheerthavarada et al., 1997) or even in the nucleus, where a P450-dependent nuclear metabolizing system has been reported (Castro et al., 1998).

Cytochrome 2E1 is the basic constituent of the MEOS system (Lasker et al., 1987) and possesses activity to oxidize besides ethanol, other alcohols such as butanol and pentanol (Morgan et al., 1982), as well as other xenobiotic compounds such as aniline, acetaminophen, carbon tetrachloride, acetone, benzene, phenol and N-nitrosodimethylamine, among others (Ingelman-Sundberg and Johansson, 1984; Koop and Tierney, 1990). This system possesses a low affinity for ethanol, with a Km of 8-10 mM, for which it is considered that in non-alcoholic individuals, its participation is only important at high tissue concentrations of the substrate. The MEOS system is the only one whose activity is significantly induced (5 - 10 fold) by the presence of ethanol or other molecules such as pyridine, acetone and pyrazole (Koop and Tierney, 1990).

Catalase

This enzyme (H_2O_2:H_2O_2 oxidoreductase; EC 1.11.1.6) is a homotetramer that possesses as prosthetic groups ferric protoporphyrin IX and $NADP^+$

(Goyal and Basak, 2010). Catalase is localized in the peroxisomes, and its main activity is the decomposition of hydrogen peroxide molecules. However, it is also highly efficient in the peroxide dependent oxidation of: nitrous, formic and hydrazoic acids, short chain aliphatic alcohols, and hydroxylamine (Schonbaum and Chance, 1976). Ethanol oxidation by catalase is coupled to the decomposition of a molecule of hydrogen peroxide, or even to the decomposition of organic peroxide. Thus, the limiting factor in the oxidation of ethanol by catalase is the availability of peroxides, for which it is considered that under normal conditions, its participation in ethanol metabolism is minimal (Cederbaum, 2012).

Non-Oxidative Ethanol Metabolism

Lange et al. (1981) showed that ethanol is capable of reacting with fatty acids to yield fatty acid ethyl esters (FAEEs) by means of an enzymatic reaction catalyzed by a fatty acid ethyl ester synthase, which does not require ATP or coenzyme A participation to catalyze the reaction (Mogelson and Lange, 1984). FAEEs generation occurs via diverse FAEE synthase enzymes (Zelner et al., 2013; Bearer, 2015) that include glutathione S-transferase, cholesterol esterase, carboxylester hydrolase, carboxylester lipase, pancreatic lipase, and lipoprotein lipase. These esters are synthesized in the endoplasmic reticulum, and transported to the plasma membrane (Cederbaum, 2012), although the mitochondria themselves are able to synthesize FAEEs in the presence of ethanol (Carrasco et al., 2007). Pancreas and liver are the organs with the highest ability to synthesize FAEEs, followed by adipose, heart, and brain (Bearer, 2015).

Organs lacking significant oxidative ethanol metabolism are frequently damaged by ethanol abuse if they have a high fatty acid ethyl ester synthetic activities and show substantial transient accumulations of fatty acid ethyl esters, such as, for example heart, pancreas and brain, among others (Laposata and Lange, 1986). Indeed, heavy drinkers exhibit high FAEE serum concentration (Doyle et al., 1994), and could serve as biomarker of either acute or chronic ethanol exposure. The mechanism of induced toxicity by FAEE is related to mitochondrial dysfunction: in pancreatic acinar cells for example, FAEEs sustain a cytosolic calcium elevation that led to necrosis (Criddle et al., 2004). This calcium overload caused loss of membrane potential with a consequent fall of ATP supply. Also, Lange and Sobel (1983) demonstrated the ability of exogenously added ethyl oleate to serve as an uncoupler of mitochondria in myocardial cells. Interestingly, inhibition of carboxyl ester lipase, a major producer of FAEEs in pancreas, partially blocked the deleterious effects of ethanol, supporting that FAEEs synthesis contributed to the mitochondrial dysfunction and cellular damage (Huang et al., 2014).

Our capacity to metabolize ethanol by this non-oxidative pathway is scarcely on the order of 0.137 nmol g^{-1} h^{-1} in homogenated human liver (Laposata and Lange, 1986), because of which it can be concluded that its participation in global ethanol metabolism (but not toxicity) is of little significance (Koop, 1989).

3. Hepatic Functions: Role of Mitochondria

The liver is considered the body largest gland (Vollmar and Menger, 2009); it is an essential organ that cannot be replaced due to the numerous functions that take in it. Among these are the nutrients uptake, storage and distribution (Cheng et al., 2015). It is composed of different types of cells; however the hepatocyte is the primary cell type that constitutes it.

The hepatocytes are vulnerable to damage due to their central role in the blood detoxification, since this process frequently exposes them to a harmful environment (Malhi et al., 2010). The drugs consumed for therapeutic purposes break down and combine in the liver, but also those toxic substances (such as abuse drugs and alcohol) known as xenobiotics which are foreign to the body, are also degraded (Auger et al., 2015).

Most of the blood flow (about 75%) comes directly from the gastrointestinal tract and spleen via the portal vein (Vollmar and Menger, 2009). This way, the blood that reaches the liver contains a lot of xenobiotics recently absorbed from the gastrointestinal tract. Given the impact that can cause the direct presence of xenobiotics in the body, the liver has developed enzymatic mechanisms to convert them into harmless or less harmful substances by hydroxylation, oxidation and conjugation reactions (Zimmerman, 1999). However, it is noteworthy that sometimes intermediary substances produced by these reactions are more harmful than the substances from which they proceed, leading to increased risk of injury.

In addition to its important detoxifying function, liver plays a central role in carbohydrates and lipids metabolism (Auger et al., 2015; Cheng et al., 2015), in the enterohepatic circulation of bile acids, in the production and secretion of many plasma proteins and in the iron and some vitamins homeostasis (Brissot and Loreal, 2015). To make these important functions, the liver needs a constant supply of energy that is mostly provided by the mitochondria. However, constant exposure of hepatic cells to harmful substances such as alcohol during the detoxification can cause alteration of some mitochondrial enzymes impacting mitochondrial metabolism and especially in the production of ATP, which in turn can be reflect in the development of a pathological liver condition (Malhi et al., 2010; Auger et al., 2015).

3.1. Mitochondria as an Independent Organelle

Each cell has a large amount of mitochondria, but especially hepatocytes are abundant in mitochondria (Basaranoglu et al., 2013). Mitochondria are organelles that have their own genome (Scheffler, 2001), which is highly susceptible to oxidative damage when exposed to ROS generation sites, due to the lack of protective histones and complete repair mechanisms (Begriche, 2009). Although nuclear genes encode the vast majority of mitochondrial proteins, 13 proteins encoded by circle mtDNA are essential for respiration and oxidative phosphorylation (Scheffler, 2001). Most of mitochondrial proteins are synthesized entirely in the cytosol and then are postranslationally imported (MacKenzie and Payne, 2007). Chaperones present in the cytosol help the correct folding and conservation of these proteins as they are targeted to specific mitochondrial surface receptors (Scheffler, 2001).

Moreover, mitochondrial morphology is not constant but varies according to the tissue to which they belong. It is important to note that recent studies indicate that mitochondria are not isolated but rather together forming a type of highly dynamic mitochondrial network in relation to its location within the cell and its movements are helped by cytoskeletal motor proteins (Scheffler, 2001; Putti et al., 2015). In addition to this, the mitochondria are constantly subjected to fission and fusion processes that are closely dependent on mitochondrial bioenergetic status (Putti et al., 2015).

It is well known that mitochondria have a prominent place in the cell being the main providers of energy as ATP. Mitochondrial functions vary in relation to the supply of substrates that they receive and the immediate cell energy needs (Putti et al., 2015). The importance of these lies in the metabolic processes occurring in them, such as electron transport and oxidative phosphorylation taking place in the inner mitochondrial membrane and whose dysfunction results in the production of ROS (Sato, 2007). Besides the above processes, Krebs cycle, urea cycle, β-oxidation and heme biosynthesis are metabolic processes that take place exclusively in mitochondria (Scheffler, 2001).

Moreover their importance in the energetic metabolism, mitochondria also have an important role in normal physiological process of cell death called apoptosis or programmed cell death (Bai and Odin, 2003). In this process regulated by the family of proteins Bcl-2, the mitochondria release cytochrome c contained in the intermembrane space to the cytosol, which initiates a cascade of enzymatic reactions that degrade cellular proteins and leads to apoptosis (Benedetti and Marucci, 1999). This process is a very important event during the normal development of an organism, as well as during development of biliary tree and hepatocytes, or in the case of pathological events as tumorogenesis (Benedetti and Marucci, 1999; Bai and Odin, 2003).

Furthermore, alcoholism is a major cause of cirrhosis and is known to be related to alterations in mitochondrial function. The mitochondrial dysfunction results in decreased ATP synthesis and increased ROS production, which can compromise the survival, function and regeneration capacity of hepatocytes, especially in pathological conditions such as cirrhosis, in which chronic damage in liver causes changes in mitochondria (Sato, 2007). In the early stages of liver chronic injury, the amount of mitochondria is reduced and an impaired mitochondrial respiration is observed. The metabolism changes and the necessary ATP is obtained predominantly from glycolysis (Nishikawa et al., 2014). However, as the disease progresses, the condition cannot be maintained and can cause liver failure and death (Nishikawa et al., 2014). Other diseases that are related to mitochondrial dysfunction and failure of liver cells regeneration are hepatocellular carcinoma, non-alcoholic steatohepatitis and insulin resistance (Sato, 2007; Auger et al., 2015). Later a more detailed description of the functional alterations caused by the deterioration of mitochondrial function is made.

3.2. Carbohydrate and Fatty Acid Catabolism

The energy required for cellular processes is obtained from the ingested food. Carbohydrates must be digested using the enzymes present in the gastrointestinal tract to be converted to monosaccharides, which are absorbed by the intestinal epithelial cells and thence passed to the hepatic portal system. Glucose is the most abundant monosaccharide found in blood, obtained from carbohydrates digestion. Once in circulation, glucose must be captured by the different tissues through transporter proteins located on cell membrane, in the case of liver, hepatocyte employs transporter GLUT2 for glucose passive income (Cohen et al., 2014). Once inside the cell and under normal conditions, glucose is metabolized to pyruvate through a series of 10 reactions known as glycolysis. In the absence of oxygen, pyruvate is converted to lactate in a process known as lactic acid fermentation (Adeva et al., 2013). In the presence of oxygen, the pyruvate formed in glycolysis comes into mitochondria where it is converted to acetyl-CoA by pyruvate dehydrogenase complex (Hiltunen et al., 2010). Acetyl-CoA is mainly channeled to the Krebs cycle (Hiltunen et al., 2010) that consists of eight reactions, which complete the oxidation of acetyl-CoA to CO_2. During these processes, the generated reduced electron carriers (NADH and $FADH_2$) pass to electron transport chain and their reoxidation will drive the biosynthesis of ATP into a reaction that consumes oxygen (Adeva et al., 2013). The acetyl-CoA metabolized in the Krebs cycle is not derived exclusively from glucose metabolism, and can also be obtained from the catabolism of fatty acids during the β-oxidation in the mitochondrial matrix and also from some amino acids metabolism (Adeva et al., 2013).

For its part, free fatty acids coming from lipids digested with help of several lipases and bile salts are also absorbed by the enterocytes. Free fatty acids reach the liver through lymphatic circulation and then into the portal circulation joined in lipoprotein particles called chylomicrons. Liver mitochondria are the primary site where β oxidation of fatty acids is performed (Begriche et al., 2006; Basaranoglu et al., 2015). The catabolism of fatty acids generally comprises three stages; the first is the activation of the fatty acids to form the corresponding acyl-CoA (Fromenty et al., 1995), which takes place in the cytosol, and in the second stage, large chain fatty acids activated must enter the mitochondria for oxidation using a transport depending on carnitine shuttles. It should be mentioned that fatty acids of medium and short chain fatty acids enter directly to the mitochondrial matrix without depending on the carnitine shuttle. In the third stage, once inside of mitochondrial matrix, the acyl-CoA formed is oxidized by a sequence of four reactions known as β-oxidation cycle that undergo oxidative removal of successive two-carbon units in the form of acetyl-CoA (Begriche et al., 2006). These four reactions are repeated until finally there are two molecules of acetyl-CoA (Begriche et al., 2009). In the case of unsaturated fatty acids oxidation additional enzymes are required and in the case of fatty acids with an odd number of carbons, the reaction sequence is the same except that at the end, a molecule of propionyl-CoA is obtained instead of the acetyl-CoA. The β oxidation is also associated to the generation of NADH and $FADH_2$ (Begriche et al., 2006; Begriche et al., 2009).

3.3. ATP Production and Oxygen Consumption

During the process of glycolysis, TCA and β-oxidation mentioned above, electron carriers in the reduced state (NADH and $FADH_2$) are produced (Scheffer, 2001; Begriche et al., 2006; Begriche et al., 2009). Now the reducing power generated when reoxidizing these molecules will be used in the electron transport chain for ATP production by oxidative phosphorylation with consequent oxygen consumption that serves as the final electron acceptor (Scheffer, 2001; Adeva et al., 2013). It is noteworthy that the process of reoxidation of the electron carriers to regenerate NAD and FAD is necessary for their reuse in other cycles of oxidation (Begriche et al., 2009).

Mitochondrial respiratory chain consists of several electron donor and acceptor molecules, arranged in four multiprotein complexes (I-IV) (Scheffer, 2001) and two mobile electrons carriers, cytochrome c and coenzyme Q_{10} (Adeva et al., 2013). Except for cytochrome c that is located in the outer surface of the inner membrane, all components of the respiratory chain are accommodated inside the inner mitochondrial membrane (Adeva et al., 2013). Each electron carriers represents a redox pair. Complex I (NADH-ubiquinone oxidoreductase) catalyze the transfer of reducing equivalents from NADH to ubiquinone (Coenzyme Q_{10}) (Adeva et al., 2013). Complex II (succinate-ubiquinone oxidoreductase) is also a component of the Krebs cycle (succinate dehydrogenase) and transports electrons from succinate to coenzyme Q_{10} (Adeva et al., 2013). Complex III (cytochrome bc 1 or ubiquinol-cytochrome *c* reductase) releases electrons from ubiquinol, the reduced form of coenzyme Q_{10} to cytochrome *c* (Adeva et al., 2013). Finally, Complex IV (cytochrome *c* oxidase) transfers electrons from cytochrome *c* to oxygen, which is reduced to produce water (Adeva et al., 2013). In complexes I, III and IV, electron transport through the components of the respiratory chain is associated with pumping of protons from the mitochondrial matrix to the intermembrane space which provides an electrochemical and proton gradient that is used by the ATP synthase also called Complex V to carry out the synthesis of ATP (Scheffer, 2001; Adeva et al., 2013). Note that in the complex II there is not proton translocation (Scheffer, 2001; Adeva et al., 2013). Binding of adenosine diphosphate (ADP) to complex V or ATP synthase induces protons to flow back from the intermembrane space into the mitochondrial matrix through a proton channel in the complex V, releasing the energy contained in the electrochemical gradient and causing the formation of ATP through ADP phosphorylation (Adeva et al., 2013).

The electron flow in the electron transport chain is controlled by the energy states of the membrane, also called phosphate potential (Sato, 2007). The electron flow is slow in a state of high energy, which means that the consumption of O_2 decreases when ATP abounds in the mitochondria (Sato, 2007). Moreover, although oxidative phosphorylation is the main source of ATP in normal cells, this energy source may change depending on the needs and stressors microenvironment (Nishikawa et al., 2014). For example, a decrease in oxygen availability reprograms mitochondria to allow the cell to generate ATP from glycolysis more than from oxidative phosphorylation (Nishikawa et al., 2014). Also, under pathological conditions such as cancer, cells can change their main source of energy production from mostly oxidative phosphorylation to glycolysis to satisfy their energy needs (Nishikawa et al., 2014).

Moreover, normally under physiological conditions, of 1-5% of the oxygen consumed during cellular respiration is not completely reduced to water, generating a certain amount of ROS (Basaranoglu et al., 2013). When any change in the constituents of the electron transport chain is present an inability to efficiently reduce O_2 to water is caused. Under these conditions, electrons can escape from the complex III, II or I and result in partial reduction of O_2, which will cause the generation of superoxide anion radical and reactive oxygen species and subsequent hydrogen peroxide and hydroxyl radical, which in turn may damage mitochondrial DNA causing a cycle of damage to components of the mitochondria (Sato, 2007). In studies conducted in hepatocytes using inhibitors of electron transport chain, it was found that the complex I and II are the main generators sites of ROS after acute exposure to ethanol (Bailey et al., 1999).

3.4. Fatty Acid Synthesis

It is well known that the biosynthesis of fatty acids occurs in the cytosol, however, a least mentioned additional fatty acids synthesis pathway takes place in the mitochondria. Some of acetyl-CoA from the oxidation of glucose is substrate for the synthesis of mitochondrial fatty acid. One of the recently recognized features of mitochondria is their ability to synthesize fatty acids in an acyl carrier protein (ACP)-dependent manner (Hiltunen et al., 2010). Besides to the function as a substrate in the synthesis of lipoic acid, the fate of products of mitochondrial fatty acid synthesis is not well known (Hiltunen et al., 2009; Hiltunen et al., 2010). Alternatively, long-chain fatty acids synthesized in mitochondria can be used for the acylation of proteins (Hiltunen et al., 2010). The synthesis of lipoic acid appears to be an essential process in mammals, deletion of lipoic acid synthase results in embryonic lethality in mice. Therefore, the conservation of alternative mitochondrial fatty acid synthesis pathway may be essential for the supply of certain types of fatty acids such as lipoic acid (Hiltunen et al., 2010).

Moreover, disturbances in the route of mitochondrial synthesis of fatty acid affects the composition of mitochondrial phospholipids, but it is unclear if this is an indirect effect of altered mitochondrial metabolism or a direct consequence of the reduced channeling of acyl groups to phospholipid synthesis (Hiltunen et al., 2010). The best-characterized function of the physiological pathway of mitochondrial fatty acid synthesis is to provide the chain octanoyl to the lipoic acid synthesis (Hiltunen et al., 2010). The synthesis of mitochondrial fatty acids has much similarity to the synthesis of bacterial fatty acids. Both use separate polypeptides that carry out individual reactions, unlike cytosolic fatty acid synthetic route of eukaryotes that carry them out by multifunctional proteins (Hiltunen et al., 2009; Hiltunen et al., 2010).

The mitochondrial pathway is best described in the yeast *S. cerevisiae*, where the deletion of any member of the mitochondrial fatty acid synthesis pathway leads to respiratory failure phenotype, lacking cytochromes and decreased lipoic acid, indicating that this pathway is essential for mitochondrial function (Hiltunen et al., 2010).

To date, the identified enzymes involved in the mitochondrial pathway of fatty acids synthesis are ACP transferase phosphopantetheine, malonyl transferase, β-ketoacyl-ACP synthase, the 3-hydroxyacyl dehydratase-thioester, enoyl thioester reductase and 3-ketoacyl reductase. Generation of malonyl-CoA is the first step in fatty acid synthesis, and the source of this compound used in the mitochondrial synthesis of fatty acids in yeast and in mitochondria of higher eukaryotes is still unknown (Hiltunen et al., 2010).

3.5. Ureagenesis

Ureagenesis refers to hepatic urea formation as a waste product of the amino acid metabolism; this is the only metabolic process that can remove nitrogen excess from the body (Deignan et al., 2008). As with carbohydrates and lipids, proteins must be broken down to simpler molecules that shape them, such as dipeptides and free amino acids, to be metabolized. Amino acids obtained from the diet that are not needed for the synthesis of other nitrogen-containing molecules and endogenous protein, can be converted to carbohydrates by removing the nitrogen. In this way a molecule remains that can be then converted to pyruvate or an intermediary of Krebs cycle to obtain energy for gluconeogenesis. The resulting ammonia is highly toxic to cells (Wraith, 2001), which must be metabolized immediately in another less toxic compound, urea, and a water-soluble compound that can be easily excreted from the body by kidneys as a urinary component (Deignan et al., 2008). Moreover, it is noteworthy that the urea cycle has not only the function of removing waste nitrogen as urea; it also carries out the *de novo* biosynthesis of the arginine amino acid (Wraith, 2001).

As mentioned above, the urea cycle is the final pathway for nitrogen metabolism. First amino acid catabolism is carried out to urea production and subsequent excretion (Foschi et al., 2015). It begins in the mitochondrial matrix and ends with the formation of urea in the cytoplasm (Wraith, 2001). The urea cycle consists on the action of mitochondrial and cytoplasmic enzymes and some transport proteins, leading to the production of urea molecules from nitrogen atoms. It consists of five consecutive enzymatic reactions that convert an ammonium nitrogen molecule, and one aspartate molecule into urea per cycle (Machado and Pinheiro da Silva, 2014). These enzymes are carbamoyl phosphate synthetase ornithine transcarbamylase, arginosuccinate synthetase, arginosuccinase, arginase and I. This process also involves enzyme producing cofactors (N-acetyl glutamate synthetase) and two transporters (citrulline and ornithine transporter 1). The urea cycle rate-limiting initial enzyme, carbamoyl phosphate synthetase 1 (CPS1), requires an allosteric activator, N-acetylglutamate (NAG) (Ah Mew and Caldovic, 2011). The formation of this unique cofactor from glutamate and acetyl CoA is catalyzed by N-acetylglutamate synthase (NAGS). An absence of NAG as a result of NAGS deficiency can compromise the flow through CPS1 and result in hyperammonemia (Ah Mew and Caldovic, 2011). The lack of any of the enzymes of the urea cycle can cause alterations in it and therefore pathologies associated with elevated ammonium such as mental retardation, coma and even death can occur (Machado and Pinheiro da Silva, 2014). Alterations in the urea cycle include a variety of genetic defects that cause deficient urea synthesis and consequent elevation of blood ammonia. These alterations are known as inborn errors of liver metabolism. Except for ornithine transcarbamylase deficiency, which is linked to the X chromosome, all disorders of the urea cycle are inherited in an autosomal recessive pattern (Deignan et al., 2009).

3.6. ROS Homeostasis

In normal conditions, most of the electrons arising from mitochondrial respiratory chain migrate along it until finally reaching the complex cytochrome c oxidase or Complex IV, where they combine with oxygen and protons to form water (Begriche et al., 2009). However, a fraction of these electrons escape from the complex I and III and reacts with the surrounding oxygen reducing it partially and resulting in the formation of superoxide anion (Begriche et al., 2009). Superoxide anion is a free radical, a molecule having an unpaired electron in the valence orbital, which is highly reactive (Cichoż-Lach and Michalak, 2014). There are reactive oxygen species (ROS) and reactive nitrogen species (RNS), the function of these reactive species is not always deleterious, since they are involved in signal transduction pathways, defense against pathogenic and regulating the expression of certain genes (Diesen and Kuo, 2011). Their impact within the cell may be either positive or negative depending on the concentration that they reach (Circu and Aw, 2010). However, the reactive species are more related to reactions with surrounding molecules (proteins, lipids, DNA) (Diesen and Kuo, 2011) which cause changes in structure and function.

To avoid such alterations cell has enzymatic (superoxide dismutase (SOD), catalase, glutathione peroxidase (GPx) and non-enzymatic (vitamin E, ascorbate, tocopherol, and glutathione (GSH)) antioxidant defense systems (Cichoż-Lach and Michalak, 2014). The most common antioxidants that can be found in hepatocytes are GSH, GPx, SOD, catalase, thioredoxin, heme oxygenase, peroxidases and some metal binding proteins (Diesen and Kuo, 2010). Superoxide anion is dismutated by mitochondrial superoxide dismutase (MnSOD) in H_2O_2, which can subsequently be detoxified in water by mitochondrial glutathione peroxidase (GPx) (Begriche et al., 2009). This enzyme needs GSH to carry out its detoxifying function, so that a deficiency of GSH can jeopardize enzyme antioxidant capacity (Begriche et al., 2009). GSH is involved in numerous redox functions, it is responsible for maintaining intracellular redox balance, when GSH, it is biologically active and during oxidative stress is oxidized to GSSG, therefore the GSH/GSSG ratio is a good indicator of the intracellular redox state (Circu and Aw, 2010). Mitochondria also have its own pool of GSH, which ensures the integrity of mitochondrial proteins and lipids (Circu and Aw, 2010). With this sequence of reactions, reactive oxygen species (ROS) are neutralized. Avoiding their capacity to cause oxidative damage to mitochondrial surrounding structures, mitochondrial dysfunction and predispose to cell death. It is noteworthy that despite the action of antioxidant systems a small amount of ROS remains without being eliminated (Begriche et al., 2009).

Generally, complex I and III produced the ROS when the electron flow is decreased and electronic carriers are mostly in the reduced state. In addition to the above, there are mitochondrial alterations that contribute to increased generation of reactive species contributing to redox imbalance in the cell and favoring an oxidative stress condition. This mitochondrial oxidative stress is caused by an imbalance between the production of mitochondrial ROS and the antioxidant mitochondrial capacity (Cichoż-Lach and Michalak, 2014). This imbalance may be due either to ROS production increase, or a mitochondrial antioxidant systems capacity (enzymatic and non-enzymatic) decrease (Cichoż-Lach and Michalak, 2014).

Moreover it is known that mitochondria are involved in alcohol metabolism and this causes oxidative stress. This is due to the imbalance in the $NADH/NAD^+$, consequence of oxidative metabolism of alcohol by aldehyde dehydrogenase and alcohol dehydrogenase that produce increased amount of NADH (see Figure 1) (Liang et al., 2013). This upregulates production of superoxide anion and therefore H_2O_2 into mitochondria and so starts an oxidative damage cascade (Liang et al., 2013).

4. Ethanol-Induced Alterations in Liver Mitochondria

In cells, the mitochondrial electron transport chain (ETC) is one of the most important sources of reactive oxygen species (ROS) (Beckman and Ames, 1998). ROS is a term that broadly describes O_2-derived free radicals such as superoxide anion ($O_2^{\cdot-}$), hydroxyl ($HO^{\cdot}$), peroxyl ($RO_2^{\cdot}$), and alkoxyl ($RO^{\cdot}$) radicals, as well as O_2-derived nonradical species such as hydrogen peroxide (H_2O_2) (Circu and Aw, 2010). Of total O_2 consumed, 1-5% is diverted to the formation of ROS, mainly at the level of complex I and complex III of ETC, and this diversion is believed to be tissue and species dependent (Turrens, 2003). Ethanol treatment executes conditions that promote ROS formation by mitochondria, effects that may be enhanced by a decrease in the mitochondrial antioxidant systems (Hoek et al., 2002). ROS generation in ETC may be promoted *in vitro* through addition of certain inhibitors of respiratory complexes, whereas some pathological situations such as cardiomyopathy (Hoek et al., 2002), hyperglycemia (Nishikawa et al.,

2000) or chronic excessive alcohol consumption may increase the *in vivo* rate of mitochondrial ROS production. Mitochondrial constituents are themselves targets of ROS and the mitochondrial management of oxidative stress as consequences both for cellular energy metabolism and for the processes that control the onset and progression of the cell death response, whether it results in apoptosis or necrosis (Luo et al., 1997). Either acute or chronic ethanol consumption produces excessive ROS, mitochondrial dysfunction and endoplasmic reticulum stress in liver (Li et al., 2014). The ethanol-dependent oxidative stress has been proven to be predominantly generated by the induction of cytochrome P450-2E1 (CYP2E1) that induce abundant ROS such as hydrogen peroxide and superoxide anion radical when metabolizing ethanol in the membrane of the endoplasmic reticulum (ER) (Lu and Cederbaum, 2008).

4.1. Redox State (NADH/NAD^+ Ratio)

Ethanol metabolism can induce modifications in liver metabolic pathways that are tightly regulated through the availability of cellular energy and through the redox state (Gutiérrez-Salinas et al., 1999). Administration of ethanol is known to readily alter the cellular redox state through its catabolism (Gutiérrez-Salinas et al., 1999).

Acute alcohol intoxication occasionally causes severe hypoglycemia, which can result in sudden death. As reviewed elsewhere (Lieber, 2000), hypoglycemia is due, in part, to the block by ethanol of hepatic gluconeogenesis, again as a consequence of the increased NADH/NAD ratio in subjects whose glycogen stores are already depleted by starvation or who have pre-existing abnormalities in carbohydrate metabolism (Lieber, 2000). The oxidant/anti-oxidant balance is quantitatively reflected in the redox state, which, in turn, is dependent upon the ratios of the interconvertible forms (reduced and oxidized) of redox couples, such as GSH/GSSG, NADH/NAD^+, NADPH/$NADP^+$, cysteine/cystine, thioredoxin red/thioredxin oxid, and glutaredoxin red/glutaredoxin oxid; however, GSH:GSSG couple is considered to be the primary intra-cellular determinant of the redox state, because it is 3 to 4 orders of magnitude more abundant than the other redox couples, and because it has a low standard redox potential (Eo=−240mV) (Rebrin and Sohal, 2008). With in vitro ethanol exposure or chronic ethanol ingestion, multiple members of the mitochondrial Thioredoxin reductase 2 (Trx2) redox circuits were oxidized, including nicotinamide adenine dinucleotide phosphate

(NADP), GSH, Trx2, Prdx, and TrxR2 (Liang et al., 2013). Extensive oxidation of the Trx 2 redox system may explain the ethanol-induced mitochondrial ROS generation and subsequent loss of critical alveolar macrophages functions such as phagocytosis (Liang et al., 2013). High levels of NADH in mitochondria can cause an increase in the number of superoxide ($O_2^{\cdot-}$) free radicals leading to the formation of hydroxyl radicals ($OH^{\cdot}$), lipid peroxidation and damage to mitochondria DNA. High levels of free radicals diminish or impair the antioxidant homeostasis, leading to tissue damage (Guo and Ren, 2010). Chronic ethanol intake enhances susceptibility to drugs toxicity, due to selective depletion of mitochondrial GSH.

4.2. Production of ROS and RNS (Electron Transport Chain, CYP2E1 and iNOS)

Chronic alcohol consumption causes numerous biochemical and biophysical changes in various organs, in which mitochondria is the primary organelle affected. Mitochondria are the target of ethanol intoxication mainly due to the increased production of reactive oxygen species/reactive nitrogen species (ROS/RNS) during ethanol metabolism (Reddy et al., 2013). The interactions between nitric oxide (NO) and mitochondrial respiration exhibits significant decrease in state 3 respiration, and respiratory control ratio, and NO-dependent inhibition of respiration (Venkatraman et al., 2003). It is well documented the importance of NO in regulating several aspects of mitochondrial function, including the formation of ROS (Ramachandran et al., 2002) and the competing reaction with oxygen in the hydrophobic phase of the mitochondrial inner membrane (Venkatraman et al., 2003). For example, NO-dependent regulation of cytochrome *c* oxidase as well as an impaired rate of adenosine triphosphate synthesis is also observed (Reddy et al., 2013). Previous reports revealed that chronic alcohol consumption inhibits complexes I and III of the mitochondrial electron transport chain and increases ROS production in liver (Zelickson et al., 2011). Superoxide ($O_2^{\cdot-}$), a reactive oxygen species, reacts directly with the NO to form peroxynitrite ($ONOO^-$) (Beckman et al., 1990) and in this way inactive it. $ONOO^-$ is extremely reactive, also oxidizes the tetrahydrobiopterin (BH_4); an important cofactor for the NOS. In the absence of BH_4, the NOS produces $O_2^{\cdot-}$ rather than NO, a process called decoupling of the NOS, managing to increase oxidative stress (Saavedra-Molina et al., 2015). The activity of respiratory enzyme complexes I and III and their linked activities are directly related to cardiolipin content

(Petrosillo et al., 2007). A study has been linked to decrease of cardiolipin in a decrease of complexes I, III and IV (Reddy et al., 2013). Decreased activity of mitochondrial complex I, III, and IV activities could be due to decreased CL content. Indeed the impairment of complex III activity due to ROS-induced cardiolipin decrease, oxidative damage may increase the electron leak from the electron transport chain, generating more superoxide radicals, which leads to mitochondrial dysfunction in alcohol-treated rats (Reddy et al., 2013). Besides another physiological factor impairs electron transport chain and NO synthesis, which is Ca^{2+} ions, reported inhibiting ATP synthesis in supraphysiological concentrations (Aguilera-Aguirre et al., 2002; Saavedra-Molina et al., 2003).

The effects of ethanol on different cells or organs are not the same, and these differences seem to depend on the NOS isoform involved. Besides, reactive α, β-unsaturated aldehydes generated as a result of lipoperoxidation could contribute to pathogenesis of lung disease, vascular disease such as atherosclerosis and other oxidative stress-related pathologies due to modification of biomolecules (Sapkota and Wyatt, 2015). Other diseases such as emphysema, asthma, Alzheimer's disease and Parkinson's disease has been linked to 4-hydroxynonenal, a highly reactive end product of lipoperoxidation (Sapkota and Wyatt, 2015). In rat neurons, 5 weeks of ethanol consumption induced an up-regulation of iNOS while nNOS-expressing neurons were down regulated (Bagyánszki et al., 2011). Same results have presented Reddy et al. (2013) in brain cortex where iNOS and nNOS mRNA and protein expression has been observed after alcohol treatment.

The microsomal ethanol-inducible cytochrome P450 (CYP) form, CYP2E1, has been shown to play a pivotal role in the pathogenesis of alcoholic liver disease, due to its potential for free radicals generation and induction of lipid peroxidation (Niemela et al., 2000). The expression of various cytochrome enzymes also occurred with the sites of acetaldehyde and lipid peroxidation-derived protein adducts. The ethanol oxidation in hepatocytes results in the formation of highly reactive aldehydes such as acetaldehyde, malondialdehyde and 4-hydroxy-2-nonenal, aldehydes that exhibit high reactivity forming adducts out (Kaur and Katyal, 2012). The covalent binding of these aldehydes to proteins interferes with protein function, but also generates antibody response (Thiele et al., 2004).

4.3. Deleterious Effects in Mitochondria (ATP Synthesis, Lipid Metabolism, Antioxidant Systems)

Loss of mitochondrial function is central to the development of oxidative stress in fatty liver disease and ethanol administration (Bailey and Cunningham, 2002). One of the earliest effects of chronic ethanol consumption on liver is an alteration in mitochondria structure in which the organelle is often enlarged and misshapen and contains disrupted cristae. Specifically, after chronic ethanol consumption there is a decrease in the rate of ATP synthesis via the oxidative phosphorylation system, implicating complex I and complex III (Gyamfi et al., 2012). Indeed, other mitochondrial functions as membrane potential ($\Delta\Psi m$), oxygen consumption and ROS production are consequences of ethanol intoxication in liver mitochondria (Gyamfi et al., 2012), as well as mitochondrial permeability transition (MPT) (El-Assai et al., 2004). Other studies include ATP-binding cassette proteins, and cytochrome P450 enzymes when alcohol is present (Jin et al., 2011). The presence of unsaturated fatty acids increases the mitochondrial injury in the development of alcohol fatty liver disease, contrary when saturated fatty acids are present in liver mitochondria (Gyamfi et al., 2012). However, studies claim that the presence of unsaturated fatty acids such as arachidonic acid (20:4) and docosahexaneoic acid (22:6), prevented fatty liver and changes to mitochondrial function such as ATP synthase (Song et al., 2008). DNA methylation, gene expression, and post-translational histone modifications were also described as damages in mouse hippocampus where maternal consumption of alcohol during pregnancy has implications to early prenatal ethanol exposure in a mouse model (Zhang et al., 2015; Marjonen et al., 2015). Perinatal ethanol toxicity alters the plasticity of neurodevelopment and the regulation of glutamatergic gene expression, also dysregulate a number of genes involved in glutamatergic signalling and synaptic plasticity, including vesicular glutamate transporter 1, complexin 1, excitatory amino acid transporters 1 and 3, and some *N*-methyl-D-aspartate (NMDA) receptor subunits (Zink et al., 2001).

4.4. Membrane Permeability Transition Pore and Apoptosis

Mitochondrial permeability transition is best defined as the collapse of the chemiosmotic gradient across the inner mitochondrial membrane mediated by opening of a large conductance pore called the mitochondrial permeability transition pore (MPTP) (Elrod and Molkentin, 2013). MPTP is characterized as increased permeability of the inner mitochondrial membrane to water and solutes, as well swelling of the mitochondria and subsequent rupture of the outer membrane (King et al., 2014). Although the specific protein components of the MPT pore remain elusive, cyclophilin D (CypD) is thought to be a key regulator of MPT pore function. Cyclophilins are conserved through all eukaryotic and even bacterial kingdoms, with most members directly binding the immunosuppressive drug cyclosporin A (CsA) (Elrod and Molkentin, 2013). King et al. (2014) observed that chronic ethanol consumption enhanced sensitivity to Ca^{2+}-dependent opening of the MPT pore in isolated rat liver mitochondria. These data suggest that increased CypD levels may predispose liver mitochondria to undergo MPT pore formation and opening response to chronic ethanol consumption. Other studies reported that chronic ethanol-mediated mitochondrial dysfunction and liver injury would be attenuated in mice lacking CypD (King et al., 2014). MPT pore has parallel observations as initiation of cell death programs, as reported (Lemasters et al., 2009) due to formation of the MPT pore causes mitochondrial depolarization and increases ROS production, which can trigger autophagy in cells (Lee et al., 2012). Autophagy is recognized as a major intracellular pathway responsible for degradation and removal of cytoplasmic proteins, lipid droplets, and damaged organelles. On this basis, mitochondria can be degraded by the autophagosomal-lysosomal pathway, i.e., mitophagy (Ashrafi and Schwarz, 2013). Indeed, it has been suggested that stimulation of autophagy reduced alcoholic steatosis and toxicity (Lin et al., 2013). Others observed cardiomyocytes isolated from mice overexpressing CypD that exhibited enhanced levels of autophagy (Carreira et al., 2010).

5. Alcoholic Liver Diseases: Steatosis (Fatty Liver); Alcoholic Hepatitis (Inflammation), Hepatic Fibrosis and Cirrhosis

There is a strong increase of diseases caused by a rising use of alcohol, and there is a clear correlation between the consumption of alcohol, the deaths induced and the capability of acquisition of drinking habits that are a problem (Sheron et al., 2008). Nevertheless, is important to note that only a minority with alcohol liver disease (ALD) develops alcohol dependence.

Several reports have been identified several risk factors such as genetic predisposition, gender, poor nutrition, obesity, and the presence of other liver diseases such as hepatitis C and complication of metabolic syndrome (Naveau et al., 1997; Forrest and Reed, 2011). ALD covers from steatosis to alcoholic steatohepatitis and cirrhosis. The physiology of the ALD includes oxidative damage; endotoxaemia which causes cell damage and even death; and the initiation of inflammatory process.

Steatosis is considered as the beginning of the ALD, which may or may not developed fibrosis, and then it come the steatohepatitis and finally the cirrhosis. Bruha et al. (2012) made a correlation between the states of the disease, taking both the steatosis and steatohepatitis as reversible and can therefore be developed for alcohol consumption and/or by metabolic syndrome. On the other hand cirrhosis is seen as irreversible and is caused by alcohol restraint, causing inflammatory processes.

The development of the disease is clear, having as final result cirrhosis. Teli et al. (1995) describe the process as dynamic. Steatosis is reversible after a period of abstinence; the steatohepatits, apparently a condition that only is related to excessive alcohol consumption, which is already developing fibrosis, is reversible but may occasionally fibrosis persist, while worsening eventually causes cirrhosis.

The disease progression is due to different factors, which together cause synergy: direct influence of alcohol on the liver, excessive caloric intake, the predisposition to obesity, among others (Shen et al., 2010). Malnutrition has been considered as another aggravating clinical issue on the development of the disease. Hard drinkers typically do not have a proper diet, which compromises the metabolism of several important nutrients such as proteins, polyunsaturated fatty acids, minerals and vitamins (Plauth et al., 2009).

Family studies have demonstrated the crucial role of genes in the propensity of development ALD. Two genes have been identified to be involved in alcohol metabolism and which mutations affect dependence on consumption. Genes coding for alcohol dehydrogenase ADH1B*1 and aldehyde dehydrogenase ALDH2*2, the first one causes a 3-fold increased risk of dependence and the second one a reduction of 10-fold (Whitfield, 1997). Inclusive Edenberg et al. (2004) has reported that alcohol dependence can also affect certain polymorphisms of GABA receptors and some other neuropeptides.

Patients with steatosis usually move towards asymptomatic, they might possibly show a slight increase in liver function and size. At steatohepatitis stage they present nausea, loss of appetite, weight loss, icterus and some liver dysfunctions (prolonged prothrombin time, hypoalbuminemia, ascites and hepatic encephalopathy). They have an increased gamma glutamyl transferase (GGT) and increased gamma globulinemia (Bruha et al., 2002).

Complications caused by cirrhosis, such as ascites, visceral bleeding and encephalopathy, are handled as ALD and other forms of chronic liver diseases. Some other complications in advanced stages of ALD (cirrhosis) include hypertension of the portal vein (Diehl, 2002), esophageal varices and hepatocellular carcinoma (Powell and Klatskin, 1968).

It is clear that inflammation plays a key role in the ALD, Kupffer cells are sensitized and this induce the secretion of pro-inflammatory intermediaries, such as TNFα and ROS, which lead to a hepatocyte necrosis and apoptosis (Tilg and Diehl, 2000). These pro-inflammatory factors have been identified to be capable of mediate some severe symptoms like anorexia, fever, fatigue, hypoalbuminemia and neutrophilia (Tilg et al., 2011).

6. Liver Injury Treatment (Mitochondrial Therapeutics)

So far, treatment for ALD includes long-term abstinence, handled with addiction services; when the disease is attached to a poor nutrition it is necessary to include of thiamine replacement. On the other hand, there is still a strong debate about the use of corticosteroids, due in part to the secondary effects of the treatment (Rambaldi et al., 2008)); finally liver transplant is considered as an option (Forrest and Reed, 2011).

Naltrexone, has been used for the prevention and treatment of ALD. It has been used as therapy of alcohol abstinence syndrome because of its anti-craving effects (Katzung and Bertram, 2007). Naltrexone, in large doses can also damage the liver. Acamprosate is used after a period of detoxification and as such is not a treatment for it, but prevents relapse by the patient in alcohol intake (Maisel et al., 2013). Adverse effects like diarrhea have been reported. It is been documented that the pentoxifiline decreases blood viscosity and the malleability of erythrocyte membranes allowing better circulation and reoxygenation of tissues (Kasper et al., 2005). Pentoxifylline (PTX) is an enzymatic inhibitor of phosphodiesterase, increases intracellular cAMP, stimulating AMPK. It is also known to be an inhibitor of TNFα (Forrest and Reed, 2011). Therefore is indicated for the treatment of liver diseases caused by alcoholism, replacing glucocorticoids. Also, authors proposed that the real beneficial effect of PTX is due to lessen risk of developing hepatorenal syndrome (Arora et al., 2011).

It has been demonstrated the good role of polyunsaturated fatty acids for treatment of ALD in animal models, possibly for their protective action by reducing oxidative and nitrosative stress (Song et al., 2008). However, there are several reports where lipids induce apoptosis; the proposed mechanism through which fatty acid induce toxicity is by translocation of bax (mitochondrial protein member of the Bcl-2 family) to the lysosomes, causing their destabilization and, producing cathepsin B, activation of nuclear factor (NFκB) and TNF-α which eventually leads to apoptosis true the activation of caspases (Feldstein et al., 2004).

Plants and plant derived products such as silymarin and resveratrol have a clear role as antioxidants in the treatment of ALD (Bishayee et al., 2010), have been documented to improve symptoms. However, their use clinically is still far from proven. The use of vitamin E, S-adenosylmethionine, betaine, N-acetyl cysteine and phlebotomy to remove iron, have also been described (Basaranoglu et al., 2013).

The obvious approach of treating with antibiotics to decrease endotoxaemia have shown little effect. On the other hand, treatments with anti-inflammatory drugs like adiponectine appear to improve ALD, presumably by increasing translation of the adiponectine receptor, which in turn reduces inflammation.

CONCLUSION

The pathological implications for excessive alcohol consumption are related to numerous diseases, as mentioned above. Alcohol consumption is considered the major source of aldehydes, protein and DNA adducts. Organs such as the liver, heart, stomach, nervous system, and lung, exposed to continuously alcohol concentration are subjected to aldehydes generation, ROS-mediated lipid peroxidation, including injuries for intracellular compartments as mitochondria. Mitochondria contribute to a high production of ROS from the electron transport chain, as well the enzymatic system of cytochrome P450. We have to add special attention on prenatal exposure to ethanol consumption during development that induces a wide spectrum of adverse effects in offspring; the most extreme of which is fetal alcohol syndrome. On the other hand, it must be considered therapeutics at the mitochondrial level for the treatment of alcohol addiction. Antioxidants or compounds with anti-inflammatory properties as curcumin, or resveratrol with cardioprotective effects has been used to prevent oxidative stress or aldehydes or adducts generation. Other studies include extracts from medicinal plants, which is promising to develop new approaches to better identify and clarify the role in alcohol-consumption. Also, the identification of possible biomarkers of susceptibility will be useful to the development of effective diagnostic therapeutic strategies.

ACKNOWLEDGMENTS

The authors appreciate the partial economic support grants from CONACYT (169093 to ASM), and CIC-UMSNH (2.16 to ASM), and UNAM (PAPIIT - IN225016 to HRR). RNC is CONACYT Postdoctoral Fellow (247328).

REFERENCES

Adeva, M; González-Lucán, M; Seco, M; Donapetry, C. (2013). Enzymes involved in l- lactate metabolism in humans. *Mitochondrion,* 13(6), 615-629.

Aguilera-Aguirre, L; González-Hernández, JC; Pérez-Vázquez, V; Ramírez, J; Clemente- Guerrero, M; Villalobos-Molina, R; Saavedra-Molina, A. (2002). Role of intramitochondrial nitric oxide in rat heart and kidney during hypertension. *Mitochondrion*, 1, 413-423.

Ah, Mew, N; Caldovic, L. (2011). N-acetylglutamate synthase deficiency: an insight into the genetics, epidemiology, pathophysiology, and treatment. *Appl Clin Genet*, 4, 127-35.

Albano, E. (2008). Oxidative mechanisms in the pathogenesis of alcoholic liver disease. *Mol Aspects Med,* 29, 9-16.

Anandatheerthavarada, HK; Addya, S; Dwivedi, RS; Biswas, G; Mullick, J; Avadhani, NG. (1997). Localization of multiple forms of inducible cytochromes P450 in rat liver mitochondria: immunological characteristics and patterns of xenobiotic substrate metabolism. *Arch Biochem Biophys,* 339, 136-150.

Anderson, P; Baumberg, B. (2006). Alcohol in Europe: A public health perspective. *Inst Arch Biochem Biophys Alcohol Studies*, London.

Arora, R; Kathuria, S; Jalandhara, N. (2011). Acute renal dysfunction in patients with alcoholic hepatitis. *World J Hepatol*, 3, 121-124.

Ashrafi, G; Schwarz, TL. (2013). The pathways of mitophagy for quality control and clearance of mitochondria. *Cell Death Differ,* 20, 31-42.

Auger, C; Alhasawi, A; Contavadoo, M; Appanna, VD. (2015). Dysfunctional mitochondrial bioenergetics and the pathogenesis of hepatic disorders. *Front Cell Dev Biol*, 3, 40. doi:10.3389/fcell.2015.00040.

Bagyánszki, M; Torfs, P; Krecsmarik, M; Fekete, E; Adriaensen, D; Van Nassauw, L; Timmermans, JP; Kroese AB. (2011). Chronic alcohol consumption induces an overproduction of NO by nNOS- and iNOS-expressing myenteric neurons in the murine small intestine. *Neurogastroenterol Motil*, 23, 237–248.

Bai, J; Odin, JA. (2003). Apoptosis and the liver: relation to autoimmunity and related conditions. *Autoimmun Rev*, 2(1), 36-42.

Bailey, SM; Cunningham, CC. (2002). Contribution of mitochondria to oxidative stress associated with alcoholic liver disease. *Free Radic Biol Med*, 32, 11-16.

Bailey, SM; Pietsch, EC; Cunningham, CC. (1999). Ethanol stimulates the production of reactive oxygen species at mitochondrial complexes I and III. *Free Radic Biol Med*, 27(7-8), 891-900.

Basaranoglu, M; Basaranoglu, G; Sentürk, H. (2013). From fatty liver to fibrosis: A tale of "second hit". *World J Gastroenterol*, 19(8), 1158-1165.

Batt, RD. (1989). Absorption, distribution, and elimination of alcohol. In: Crow KE, Batt RD, Eds. Human Metabolism of Alcohol, Vol. I: Pharmacokinetics, Medicolegal Aspects, and General Interest. Boca Raton, FL. CRC Press, 3-8.

Battelli, F; Stern, L. (1909). L'alcoolase dans les tissus animaux, C. R. *Seances Soc Biol Fil,* 67, 419–421.

Bearer, CF. (2015). A short history of fatty acid ethyl esters. *Alcohol Clin Exp Res,* 39, 413-415.

Beckman KB, Ames BN. (1998). The free radical theory of aging matures. *Phys Rev,* 78, 547-581.

Beckman, JS; Beckman, TW; Chen, J; Marshall, PA; Freeman, BA. (1990). Apparent hydroxyl radical production by peroxynitrite: Implications for endothelial injury from nitric oxide and superoxide. *Proc Natl Acad Sci USA,* 87, 1620-1624.

Begriche, K; Knockaert, L; Massart, J; Robin, MA; Fromenty, B. (2009). Mitochondrial dysfunction in nonalcoholic steatohepatitis (NASH): are there drugs able to improve it? *Drug Discov Today Dis Mech*, 6, e11-e23.

Benedetti, A; Marucci, L. (1999). The significance of apoptosis in the liver. *Liver,* 19(6), 453-63.

Best, CH; Hartroft, WS; Lucas, CC; Ridout, JH. (1949). Liver damage produced by feeding alcohol or sugar and its prevention by choline. *Br Med J,* 2, 1001-1006.

Bishayee, A; Darvesh, AS; Politis, T; McGory, R. (2010). Resveratrol and liver disease: from bench to bedside and community. *Liver Int*, 30, 1103-1114.

Brissot, P; Loreal, O. (2015). Iron metabolism and related genetic diseases: a cleared land, keeping mysteries. *J Hepatol*, 15, 00742-00744.

Bruha, R; Dvorak, K; Petrtyl, J. (2012). Alcoholic liver disease. *World J Hepatol,* 4(3), 81- 90.

Carrasco, MP; Jimenez-Lopez, JM; Segovia, JL; Marco C. (2007). Effects of ethanol on the remodeling of neutral lipids and phospholipids in brain mitochondria and microsomes. *Neurochem Int,* 50, 858-865.

Carreira, RS; Lee, Y; Ghochani, M; Gustafsson, AB; Gottlieb, RA. (2010). Cyclophilin D is required for mitochondrial removal by autophagy in cardiac cells. *Autophagy*, 6, 462-472.

Castro, GD; Delgado de Layño, AMA; Castro, JA. (1998). Liver nuclear ethanol metabolizing system (NEMS) producing acetaldehyde and 1-hydroxyethyl free radicals. *Toxicology,* 129, 137-144.

Cederbaum, AI. (2012). Alcohol metabolism. *Clin Liver Dis,* 16, 667-685.

Cheng, Y-S; Seibert, O; Klöting, N; Dietrich, A; Straßburger, K; Fernández-Veledo, S; Vendrel, JJ; Zorzano, A; Blüher, M; Herzig, S; Diaz, MB; Teleman, AA. (2015). PPP2R5C Couples Hepatic Glucose and Lipid Homeostasis. *PLoS Genetics,* 11(10), e1005561.

Cichoż-Lach, H; Michalak, A. (2014). Oxidative stress as a crucial factor in liver diseases. *World J Gastroenterol*, 20(25), 8082-8091.

Circu, ML; Aw, TY. (2010). Reactive oxygen species, cellular redox systems, and apoptosis. *Free Radic Biol Med,* 48(6), 749-762.

Cohen, M; Kitsberg, D; Tsytkin, S; Shulman, M; Aroeti, B; Nahmias, Y. (2014). Live imaging of GLUT2 glucose-dependent trafficking and its inhibition in polarized epithelial cysts. *Open Biol,* 4, 140091.

Crabb, DW; Bosron, WF; Li, TK. (1987). Ethanol metabolism. *Pharmacol Ther,* 34, 59-73.

Criddle, DN; Raraty, MG; Neoptolemos, JP; Tepikin, AV; Petersen, OH; Sutton, R. (2004). Ethanol toxicity in pancreatic acinar cells: mediation by nonoxidative fatty acid metabolites. *Proc Natl Acad Sci USA,* 101, 10738-10743.

Deignan, JL; Cederbaum, SD; Grody, WW. (2008). Contrasting features of urea cycle disorders in human patients and knockout mouse models. *Mol Genet Metab*, 93(1), 7-14.

Diehl, AM. (2002). Liver disease in alcohol abusers: clinical perspective. *Alcohol*, 27, 7-11.

Diesen, DL; Kuo, PC. (2010). Nitric oxide and redox regulation in the liver: Part I. General considerations and redox biology in hepatitis. *J Surg Res*, 162(1), 95-109.

Doyle, KM; Bird, DA; al-Salihi, S; Hallaq, Y; Cluette-Brown, JE; Goss, KA; Laposata, M. (1994). Fatty acid ethyl esters are present in human serum after ethanol ingestion. *J Lipid Res,* 35, 428-437.

Edenberg, HJ; Dick, DM; Xuei, X; Tian, H; Almasy, L; Bauer, LO; Crowe, RR; Goate, A; Hesselbrock, V; Jones, K; Kwon, J; Li, TK; Nurnberger, JI; O'Connor, SJ; Reich, T; Rice, J; Schuckit, MA; Porjesz, B; Foroud, T; Begleiter, H. (2004). Variations in GABRA2, encoding the alpha 2 subunit of the GABA(A) receptor, are associated with alcohol dependence and with brain oscillations. *Am J Hum Genet*, 74, 705-714.

Elamin, EE; Mascle, AA; Dekker, J; Jonkers, DM. (2013). Ethanol metabolism and its effects on the intestinal epithelial barrier. *Nutrition Rev*, 71, 483-489.

El-Assal, O; Hong, F; Kim, WH; Radaeva, S; Gao, B. (2004). IL-6-deficient mice are susceptible to ethanol-induced hepatic steatosis: IL-6 protects against ethanol- induced oxidative stress and mitochondrial permeability transition in the liver. *Cell Mol Immunol*, 1(3), 205-211.

Elrod, JW; Molkentin, JD. (2013). Physiologic functions of cyclophilin D and the mitochondrial permeability transition pore. *Circ J*, 77, 1111-1122.

Feldstein, AE; Werneburg, NW; Canbay, A; Guicciardi, ME; Bronk, SF; Rydzewski, R; Burgart, LJ; Gores, GJ. (2004). Free fatty acids promote hepatic lipotoxicity by stimulating TNF-alpha expression via a lysosomal pathway. *Hepatology*, 40(1), 185-194.

Forrest, E; Reed, E. (2011). Alcohol and the liver. *Medicine*, 39, 532-535.

Foschi, FG; Morelli, MC; Savini, S; Dall'Aglio, AC; Lanzi, A; Cescon, M; Ercolani, G; Cucchetti, A; Pinna, A. D; Stefanini, GF. (2015). Urea cycle disorders: a case report of a successful treatment with liver transplant and a literature review. *World J Gastroenterol*, 21(13), 4063-4068.

Fromenty, B; Pessayre, D. (1995). Inhibition of mitochondrial beta-oxidation as a mechanism of hepatotoxicity. *Pharmc Ther*, 67(1), 101-154.

González-Duarte, R; Albalat, R. (2005). Mergin protein, gene and genomic data: The evolution of the MDR-ADH family. *Heredity*, 95(3), 184-197.

Gotoh, Y; Sumimoto, H; Minakami, S. (1990). Formation of 20-oxoleukotriene B4 by an alcohol dehydrogenase isolated from human neutrophils. *Biochim Biophys Acta,* 1043, 52-56.

Goyal, MM; Basak, A. (2010). Human catalase: looking for complete identity. *Protein Cell,* 1, 888-897.

Guo, R; Ren, J. (2010). Alcohol and Acetaldehyde in Public Health: From Marvel to Menace. *Int J Environ Res Public Health,* 7, 1285-1301.

Guo, R; Ren, J. (2010). Alcohol and acetaldehyde in public health: From marvel to menace. *Int J Environ Res Public Health*, 7, 1285-1301.

Gutiérrez-Salinas, JG; Miranda-Garduño, L; Trejo-Izquierdo, E; Díaz-Muñoz, M; Vidrio, S; Morales-González, JA; Hernández-Muñoz R. (1999). Redox state and energy metabolism during liver regeneration. *Biochem Pharmacol*, 58, 1831-1839.

Gyamfi, D; Everitt, HE; Tewfik, I; Clemens, DL; Patel, VB. (2012). Hepatic mitochondrial dysfunction induced by fatty acids and ethanol. *Free Radic Biol Med*, 53, 2131- 2145.

Han, CL; Liao, CS; Wu, CW; Hwong CL; Lee, AR; Yin, SJ. (1998). Contribution to first- pass metabolism of ethanol and inhibition by ethanol for retinol oxidation in human alcohol dehydrogenase family--implications for etiology of fetal alcohol syndrome and alcohol-related diseases. *Eur J Biochem,* 254, 25-31.

Herd, D. (1992). Ideology, history and changing models of liver cirrhosis epidemiology. *Br J Addict,* 87, 1113-1126.

Hernández-Tobías, A; Julián-Sánchez, A; Piña, E; Riveros-Rosas, H. (2011). Natural alcohol exposure: Is ethanol the main substrate for alcohol dehydrogenases in animals? *Chemico-Biol Interact,* 191, 14-25.

Hiltunen, JK; Schonauer, MS; Autio, KJ; Mittelmeier, TM; Kastaniotis, AJ; Dieckmann, CL. (2009). Mitochondrial Fatty Acid Synthesis Type II: More than Just Fatty Acids. *J Biol Chem*, 284(14), 9011-9015.

Hiltunen, JK; Chen, Z; Haapalainen, AM; Wierenga, RK; Kastaniotis, AJ. (2010). Mitochondrial fatty acid synthesis-an adopted set of enzymes making a pathway of major importance for the cellular metabolism. *Prog Lipid Res,* 49(1), 27-45.

Hoek, JB; Cahill, A; Pastorino, JG. (2002). Alcohol and mitochondria. A dysfunctional relationship. *Gastroenterology*, 122, 2049-2063.

Holford, NH. (1987). Clinical pharmacokinetics of ethanol. *Clin Pharmacokinet,* 13, 273- 292.

Huang, W; Booth, DM; Cane, MC; Chvanov, M; Javed, MA; Elliott, VL; Armstrong, JA; Dingsdale, H; Cash, N; Li, Y; Greenhalf, W; Mukherjee, R; Kaphalia, BS; Jaffar, M; Petersen, OH; Tepikin, AV; Sutton, R; Criddle, DN. (2014). Fatty acid ethyl ester synthase inhibition ameliorates ethanol-induced Ca^{2+}-dependent mitochondrial dysfunction and acute pancreatitis. *Gut,* 63, 1313-1324.

Ingelman-Sundberg, M; Johansson, I. (1984). Mechanisms of hydroxyl radical formation and ethanol oxidation by ethanol-inducible and other forms of rabbit liver microsomal cytochromes P-450. *J Biol Chem,* 259, 6447-6458.

Jin, M; Arya, P; Patel, K; Singh, B; Silverstein, PS; Bhat, HK; Kumar, A; Kumar, S. (2011). Effect of alcohol on drug efflux protein and drug metabolic enzymes in U937 macrophages. *Alcohol Clin Exp Res,* 35(1), 132-139.

Jones, W; Bianchi, K. (2015). Aerobic glycolysis: beyond proliferation. *Front Immunol*, 15(6), 227.

Kasper, DL; Braunwald, E; Fauci, AS; Hauser, SL; Longo, DL; Jameson, JL. (2005). Principles of Internal Medicine, 16th Edition McGraw-Hill Medical Publishing Division, 2, 607.

Katzung, Bertram G. 2007. "31. Opioid Analgesics & Antagonists". Basic & Clinical Pharmacology (9 edition). McGraw-Hill.

Kaur, I; Katyal, A. (2012). Immunoproteomic identification of biotransformed self-proteins from the livers of female Balb/c mice following chronic ethanol administration. *Proteomics*, 12, 2036-2044.

King, AL; Swain, TM; Mao, Z; Udoh, US; Oliva, CR; Betancourt, AM; Griguer, CE; Crowe, DR; Lesort, M; Bailey, SM. (2014). Involvement of the mitochondrial permeability transition pore in chronic ethanol-mediated liver injury in mice. *Am J Physiol Gastrointest Liver Physiol*, 306, G265-G277.

Knapp, VJ. (1998). The medical response to rising alcohol consumption in 18th- and 19th- century Europe. *Nutr Health,* 12, 163-179.

Koop, DR; Tierney, DJ. (1990). Multiple mechanisms in the regulation of ethanol-inducible cytochrome P450IIE1. *BioEssays,* 12, 429-435.

Koop, DR. (1989). Minor pathways of ethanol metabolism. In Crow KE, Batt RD, Eds. Human Metabolism of Alcohol, Vol. II: Regulation, Enzymology, and Metabolites of Ethanol. Boca Raton, FL: CRC Press, 133-145.

Ladenstein, L; Winberg, JO; Benach, J. (2008). Medium- and short-chain dehydrogenase/reductase gene and protein families: Structure-function relationships in short-chain alcohol dehydrogenases, *Cell Mol Life Sci,* 65, 3918-3935.

Lange, LG; Bergman, SR; Sobel, BE. (1981). Identification of fatty acid ethyl esters as products of rabbit myocardial ethanol metabolism. *J Biol Chem,* 256, 12968-12973.

Lange, LG; Sobel, BE. (1983). Mitochondrial dysfunction induced by fatty acid ethyl esters, myocardial metabolites of ethanol. *J Clin Invest,* 72, 724-731.

Laposata, EA; Lange, LG. (1986). Presence of nonoxidative ethanol metabolism in human organs commonly damaged by ethanol abuse. *Science,* 231, 497-499.

Lasker, JM; Raucy, J; Kubota, S; Bloswick, BP; Black, M; Lieber, CS. (1987). Purification and characterization of human liver cytochrome P-450-ALC. *Biochem Biophys Res Commun,* 148, 232-238.

Lee, J; Giordano, S; Zhang, J. (2012). Autophagy, mitochondria and oxidative stress: cross- talk and redox signalling. *Biochem J*, 441, 523-540.

Lelbach, WK. (1974). Organic pathology related to volume and patterns of alcohol use. *Res Adv Alcohol Drug Problems,* 1, 93-198.

Lemasters, JJ; Theruvath, TP; Zhong, Z; Nieminen, AL. (2009). Mitochondrial calcium and the permeability transition in cell death. *Biochim Biophys Acta,* 1787, 1395- 1401.

Lenaz, G; Baracca, A; Carelli, V; D'Aurelio, M; Sgarbi, G; Solaini, G. (2004). Bioenergetics of mitochondrial diseases associated with mtDNA mutations. *Biochim Biophys Acta*, 1658(1-2), 89-94.

Li, ZL; Dong, XZ; Wang, DX; Dong, RH; Guo, TT; Sun, Y; Liu, P. (2014). Effect of oligosaccharide esters and polygalaxanthone Ill from Polygala tenuifolia willd towards cytochrome P450. *Zhongguo Zhong Yao Za Zhi*, 39(22):4459-63.

Liang, Y; Harris, FL; Jones, DP; Brown LAS. (2013). Alcohol induces mitochondrial redox imbalance in alveolar macrophages. *Free Radic Biol Med*, 65, 1427-1434.

Lieber, CS. (2000). Alcoholic liver disease: new insights in pathogenesis lead to new treatments. *J Hepatology*, 32(suppl.1), 113-128.

Lieber, CS; DeCarli, LM. (1968). Ethanol oxidation by hepatic microsomes: adaptive increase after ethanol feeding. *Science,* 162, 917-918.

Lieber, CS; Jones, DP; DeCarli, LM. (1965). Effects of prolonged ethanol intake: production of fatty liver despite adequate diets. *J Clin Invest,* 44, 1009-1021.

Lieber, CS. (2004). The discovery of the microsomal ethanol oxidizing system and its physiologic and pathologic role. *Drug Metab Rev,* 36, 511-529.

Lieber, CS. (2005). Metabolism of alcohol. *Clin Liver Dis*, 9, 1-35.

Lievens, D; Vander Laenen, F; Christiaens, J. (2014). Public spending for illegal drug and alcohol treatment in hospitals: an EU cross-country comparison. *Subst Abuse Treat Prev Policy,* 9, 26.

Lin, CW; Zhang, H; Li, M; Xiong, X; Chen, X; Chen, X; Dong, XC; Yin, XM. (2013). Pharmacological promotion of autophagy alleviates steatosis and injury in alcoholic and non-alcoholic fatty liver conditions in mice. *J Hepatol*, 58, 993-999.

Lu, Y; Cederbaum, AI. (2008). CYP2E1 and oxidative liver injury by alcohol. *Free Radic Biol Med*, 44, 724-738.

Luo, X; Pitkänen, S; Kassovska-Bratinova, S; Robinson, BH; Lehotay, DC. (1997). Excessive formation of hydroxyl radicals and aldehydic lipid peroxidation products in cultured skin fibroblasts from patients with complex I deficiency. *J Clin Invest*, 99, 2877-2882.

Machado, MC; Pinheiro da Silva, F. (2014). Hyperammonemia due to urea cycle disorders: a potentially fatal condition in the intensive care setting. *J Intensive Care*, 132(1), 22.

MacKenzie, JA; Payne, RM. (2007). Mitochondrial protein import and human health and disease. *Biochim Biophys Acta*, 1772(5), 509-523.

Maisel, NC1; Blodgett, JC; Wilbourne, PL; Humphreys, K; Finney, JW. (2013). Meta- analysis of naltrexone and acamprosate for treating alcohol use disorders: when are these medications most helpful? *Addiction*, 108(2), 275-293.

Malhi, H; Guicciardi, ME; Gores, GJ. (2010). Hepatocyte death: a clear and present danger. *Physiol Rev*, 90(3), 1165-1194.

Mann, RE; Smart, RG; Govoni, R. (2003). The Epidemiology of Alcoholic Liver Disease, *Alcohol Res Health,* 27, 210-219.

Mardh, G; Vallee, BL. (1986). Human class I alcohol dehydrogenases catalyze the interconversion of alcohols and aldehydes in the metabolism of dopamine. *Biochemistry,* 25, 7279-7282.

Marjonen, H; Sierra, A; Nyman A; Rogojin, V; Grohn, O; Linden, AM; Hautaniemi, S; Kaminen-Ahola, N. (2015). Early maternal alcohol consumption alters hippocampal DNA methylation, gene expression and volume in a mouse model. *PLoS One*, 10(5), e0124931.

McEvily, AJ; Holmquist, B; Auld, DS; Vallee, BL. (1988). 3 beta-Hydroxy-5 beta-steroid dehydrogenase activity of human liver alcohol dehydrogenase is specific to gamma- subunits. *Biochemistry,* 27, 4284-4288.

Mello, T; Ceni, E; Surrenti, C; Galli, A. (2008). Alcohol induced hepatic fibrosis: Role of acetaldehyde. *Mol Aspects Med,* 29, 17-21.

Mogelson, S; Lange, LG. (1984). Nonoxidative ethanol metabolism in rabbit myocardium: Purification to homogeneity of fatty acyl ethyl ester synthase. *Biochemistry,* 23, 4075-4081.

Morgan, ET; Koop, DR; Coon, MJ. (1982). Catalytic activity of cytochrome P-450 isozyme 3a isolated from liver microsomes of ethanol-treated rabbits. *J Biol Chem,* 257, 13951-13957.

Nagamani, SCS; Erez, A; Lee, B. (2011). Argininosuccinate Lyase Deficiency. In: Pagon RA, Adam MP, Ardinger HH, et al., editors. GeneReviews® [Internet]. Seattle (WA): University of Washington, Seattle; 1993-2015. Available from: http://www.ncbi.nlm.nih. gov/ books/NBK51784/

Naveau, S; Giraud, V; Borotto, E; Aubert, A; Capron, F; Chaput, JC. (1997). Excess weight risk factor for alcoholic liver disease. *Hepatology*, 25, 108-111.

Nebert, DW; Wikvall, K; Miller, WL. (2013). Human cytochromes P450 in health and disease. *Philos Trans R Soc Lond B Biol Sci*, 368, 20120431.

Nelson, DR; Kamataki, T; Waxman, DJ; Guengerich, FP; Estabrook, RW; Feyereisen, R; Gonzalez, FJ; Coon, MJ; Gunsalus, IC; Gotoh, O; Okuda, K; Nebert, DW. (1993). The P450 superfamily: Update on new sequences, gene mapping, accession numbers, early trivial names of enzymes, and nomenclature. *DNA Cell Biol*, 12, 1- 51.

Niemela, O; Parkkila, S; Juvonen, RO; Viitala, K; Gelboin, HV; Pasanen, M. (2000). Cytochromes P450 2A6, 2E1, and 3A and production of protein-aldehyde adducts in the liver of patients with alcoholic and non-alcoholic liver diseases. *J Hepatol*, 33, 893-901.

Nikelly, AG. (1994). Alcoholism: Social as well as psycho-medical problem -- The missing "big picture". *J Alcohol Drug Educ,* 39, 1-12.

Nishikawa, T; Bellance, N; Damm, A; Bing, H; Zhu, Z; Handa, K; Yovchev, MI; Sehgal, V; Moss, TJ; Oertel, M; Ram, PT; Pipinos, II; Soto-Gutierrez, A; Fox, I. J; Nagrath, D. (2014). A switch in the source of ATP production and a loss in capacity to perform glycolysis are hallmarks of hepatocyte failure in advance liver disease. *J Hepatol*, 60(6), 1203-1211.

Nishikawa, T; Edelstein, D; Du, XL; Yamagishi, SI; Matsumura, T; Kaneda, Y; Yorek, MA; Beebe, D; Oates, PJ; Hammes, H-P; Giardino, I;

Brownlee, M. (2000). Normalizing mitochondrial superoxide production blocks three pathways of hyperglycaemic damage. *Nature,* 404, 787-790.

Orme-Johnson, WH; Ziegler, DM. (1965). Alcohol mixed function oxidase activity of mammalian liver microsomes. *Biochem Biophys Res Commun,* 21, 78-82.

Petrosillo, G; Portincasa, P; Grattagliano, I; Casanova, G; Matera M, Ruggiero, FM; Ferri, D; Paradies, G. (2007). Mitochondrial dysfunction in rat with nonalcoholic fatty liver. Involvement of complex I, reactive oxygen species and cardiolipin. *Biochim Biophys Acta,* 1767, 1260-1267.

Phillips, R. (2014). Alcohol: a history, The University of North Carolina Press, USA.

Plauth, M; Cabré, E; Campillo, B; Kondrup, J; Marchesini, G; Schütz, T; Shenkin, A; Wendon, J. (2009). ESPEN Guidelines on Parenteral Nutrition: hepatology. *Clin Nutr*, 28, 436-444.

Powell, WJ; Klatskin, G. (1968). Duration of survival in patients with Laennec's cirrhosis. Influence of alcohol withdrawal, and possible effects of recent changes in general management of the disease. *Am J Med*, 44, 406-420.

Putti, R; Sica, R; Migliaccio, V; Lionetti, L. (2015). Diet impact on mitochondrial bioenergetics and dynamics. *Front Physiol,* 6, 109.

Ramachndran, A; Levonen, AI; Brookes, PS; Ceaser, E; Shiva, S; Barone, MC; Darley- Usmar, VM. (2002). Mitochondria, nitric oxide, and cardiovascular dysfunction. *Free Radic Biol Med*, 33, 1465-1474.

Rambaldi, A; Saconato, HH; Christensen, E; Thorlund, K; Wetterslev, J; Gluud, C. (2008). Systematic review: glucocorticosteroids for alcoholic hepatitis--a Cochrane Hepato- Biliary Group systematic review with meta-analyses and trial sequential analyses of randomized clinical trials. *Aliment Pharmacol Ther*, 27, 1167-1178.

Rebrin, I; Sohal, RS. (2008). Pro-oxidant shift in glutathione redox state during aging. *Adv Drug Deliv Rev*, 60, 1545-1552.

Reddy, DV; Padmavathi, P; Kavitha, G; Saradamma, B; Varadacharyulu, N. (2013). Alcohol-induced oxidative/nitrosative stress alters brain mitocondrial membrane properties. *Mol Cell Biochem*, 375, 39-47.

Rehm, J; Mathers, C; Popova, S; Thavorncharoensap, M; Teerawattananon, Y; Patra, J. (2009). Alcohol and Global Health 1: Global burden of disease and injury and economic cost attributable to alcohol use and alcohol-use disorders. *Lancet,* 373, 2223-2233.

Reid, MF; Fewson, CA. (1994). Molecular characterization of microbial alcohol dehydrogenases. *Crit Rev Microbiol*, 20, 13-56.

Riveros-Rosas, H; Julián-Sánchez, A; Piña, E. (1997). Enzymology of ethanol and acetaldehyde metabolism in mammals. *Arch Med Res,* 28, 453-471.

Riveros-Rosas, H; Julián-Sánchez, A; Villalobos-Molina, R; Pardo, JP; Piña, E. (2003). Diversity, taxonomy and evolution of medium-chain dehydrogenase/reductase superfamily. *Eur J Biochem,* 270, 3309-3334.

Room, R; Babor, T; Rehm, J. (2005). Alcohol and public health. *Lancet,* 365, 519-530.

Rubin, E; Hutterer, F; Lieber, CS. (1968). Ethanol increases hepatic smooth endoplasmic reticulum and drug metabolizing enzymes. *Science,* 159, 1469-1470.

Saavedra-Molina, A; Ramírez-Emiliano, J; Clemente-Guerrero, M; Pérez-Vázquez, V; Aguilera-Aguirre, L; González-Hernández, JC. (2003). Mitochondrial nitric oxide inhibits ATP synthesis. Effect of free calcium in rat heart. *Amino Acids*, 24: 95-102.

Saavedra-Molina, A; Salgado-Garciglia, R; Noriega-Cisneros, R; Esquivel-Gutiérrez, ER; Manzo-Avalos, S; Cortés-Rojo, C; Montoya-Pérez, R. (2015). Oxidative stress in diabetes and hypertension treated with alternative therapy of medicinal plants. In: A. Catalá ed. *Reactive Oxygen Species, Lipid Peroxidation and Protein Oxidation*. Nova Science Publishers, Inc. NY. USA, 205-217.

Sapkota, M; Wyatt, TA. (2015). Alcohol, aldehydes, adducts and airways. *Biomolecules*, 5, 2987-3008.

Sato, N. (2007). Central role of mitochondria in metabolic regulation of liver pathophysiology. *J Gastroenterol Hepatol*, 22 Suppl 1, S1-S6.

Scheffler, IE. (2001). Mitochondria make a come back. *Adv Drug Deliv Rev*, 49(1-2), 3-26.

Schonbaum, GR; Chance, B. (1976). Catalase. In Boyer PD, Ed. The enzymes. Vol. XIII: Oxidation-reduction, part C: Dehydrogenases (II), Oxidases (II), Hydrogen peroxide cleavage, Third ed. New York: Academic Press, 363-408.

Sellin, S; Holmquist, B; Mannervik, B; Vallee, BL. (1991). Oxidation and reduction of 4- hydroxyalkenals catalyzed by isozymes of human alcohol dehydrogenase. *Biochemistry,* 30, 2514-2518.

Shelmet, JJ; Reichard, GA; Skutches, CL; Hoeldtke, RD; Owen, OE; Boden, G. (1988). Ethanol causes acute inhibition of carbohydrate, fat, and protein oxidation and insulin resistance. *J Clin Invest,* 81, 1137-1145.

Shen, Z; Li, Y; Yu, C; Shen, Y; Xu, L; Xu, C; Xu, G. (2010). A cohort study of the effect of alcohol consumption and obesity on serum liver enzyme levels. *Eur J Gastroenterol Hepatol*, 22, 820-825.

Sheron, N; Olsen, N; Gilmore, I. (2008). An evidence-based alcohol policy. *Gut*, 57(10), 1341-1344.

Singer, M. (1986). Toward a political-economy of alcoholism: the missing link in the anthropology of drinking. *Soc Sci Med*, 23, 113-130.

Song, BJ; Moon, KH; Olsson, NU; Salem, Jr. N. (2008). Prevention of alcohol fatty liver and mitochondrial dysfunction in the rat by long-chain polyunsaturated fatty acids. *J Hepatol*, 49, 262-273.

Staab, CA; Hellgren, M; Hoog, JO. (2008). Medium- and short-chain dehydrogenase/reductase gene and protein families: Dual functions of alcohol dehydrogenase 3: implications with focus on formaldehyde dehydrogenase and S- nitrosoglutathione reductase activities. *Cell Mol Life Sci*, 65, 3950-3960.

Svensson, S; Some, M; Lundsjo, A; Helander, A; Cronholm, T; Hoog, JO. (1999). Activities of human alcohol dehydrogenases in the metabolic pathways of ethanol and serotonin. *Eur J Biochem,* 262, 324-329.

Teli, MR; Day, CP; Burt, AD; Bennett, MK; James, OF. (1995). Determinants of progression to cirrhosis or fibrosis in pure alcoholic fatty liver. *Lancet,* 346, 987- 990.

Thiele, GM; Freeman, TL; Klassen, LW. (2004). Immunologic mechanisms of alcoholic liver injury. *Semin Liver Dis,* 24, 273-287.

Tilg, H; Diehl, AM. (2000). Cytokines in alcoholic and nonalcoholic steatohepatitis. *N Engl J Med*, 343(20), 1467-76.

Tilg, H; Moschen, AR; Kaneider, NC. (2011). Pathways of liver injury in alcoholic liver disease. *J Hepatol*, 55(5), 1159-1161.

Turrens, JF. (2003). Mitochondrial formation of reactive oxygen species. *J Physiol*, 552, 335-344.

Venkatraman, A; Shiva, S; Davis, AJ; Bailey, SM; Brookes, PS; Darley-Usmar, VM. (2003). Chronic alcohol consumption increases the sensitivity of rat liver mitochondrial respiration to inhibition by nitric oxide. *Hepatology*, 38, 141-147.

Vollmar B, Menger MD. (2009). The hepatic microcirculation: mechanistic contributions and therapeutic targets in liver injury and repair. *Physiol Rev*, 89, 1269–1339.

Watson, PE. (1989). Total body water and blood alcohol levels: updating the fundamentals. In Crow KE, Batt RD, Eds. Human metabolism of alcohol, Vol. I: Pharmacokinetics, medico legal aspects, and general interest. Boca Raton, FL: CRC Press, 41-58.

Whitfield, JB. (1997). Meta-analysis of the effects of alcohol dehydrogenase genotype on alcohol dependence and alcoholic liver disease. *Alcohol Alcohol*, 32, 613-619.

WHO. 2011. Global status reports on alcohol and health. World Health Organization, Geneva, Switzerland.

Wraith, JE. (2001). Ornithine carbamoyltransferase deficiency. *Arch Dis Child,* 84(1), 84- 88.

Yao, CT; Lai, CL; Hsieh, HS; Chi, CW; Yin, SJ. (2010). Establishment of steady-state metabolism of ethanol in perfused rat liver: the quantitative analysis using kinetic mechanism-based rate equations of alcohol dehydrogenase. *Alcohol,* 44, 541-551.

Zelickson, BR; Benavides, GA; Johnson, MS; Chacko, BK; Venkatraman, A; Landar, A; Betancourt, AM; Bailey, SM; Darley-Usmar, VM. (2011). Nitric oxide and hypoxia exacerbate alcohol-induced mitochondrial dysfunction in hepatocytes. *Biochim Biophys Acta,* 1807, 1573-1582.

Zelner, I; Matlow, JN; Natekar, A; Koren, G. (2013). Synthesis of fatty acid ethyl esters in mammalian tissues after ethanol exposure: a systematic review of the literature. *Drug Metab Rev*, 45, 277-299.

Zhang, CR; Ho, MF; Vega, MF; Burne, TH; Chong, S. (2015). Prenatal ethanol exposure alters adult hippocampal VGLUT2 expression with concomitant changes in promoter DNA methylation, H3K4 trimethylation and miR-467b-5p levels. *Epigenetics Chromatin*, Doi: 10.1186/s13072-015.0032-6.

Zink, M; Ferbert, T; Frank, ST; Seufert, P; Gebicke-Haerter, PJ; Spanagel, R. (2011). Perinatal exposure to alcohol disturbs spatial learning and glutamate transmission- related gene expression in the adult hippocampus. *Eur J Neurosci*, 34(3), 457-468.

Zimmerman, HJ. (1999). Drug-induced liver disease. In: Zimmerman, HJ, ed. Hepatotoxicity: The Adverse Effects of Drugs and Other Chemicals on the Liver. 2nd ed. Philadelphia, PA: Lippincott Williams & Wilkins; 11-12.

EDITOR'S CONTACT INFORMATION

Dr. Gerond Lake-Bakaar, MD, PhD
Associate Professor of Medicine
Beth Israel Deaconess Medical Center
Harvard Medical School, Director, Liver Tumor Center
110 Francis Street, LMOB 7A, Boston, MA 02215
Email: glakebak@verizon.net

INDEX

A

Abraham, 107
abuse, 9, 74, 89, 90, 97
access, 86
accounting, 81
acetaldehyde, 3, 4, 5, 6, 9, 11, 14, 20, 24, 29, 33, 65, 66, 110, 111, 112
acetone, 13
acid, vii, 1, 4, 6, 8, 27, 37, 38, 39, 41, 45, 65, 66, 68, 69, 73, 75, 102, 110
acidosis, 14
acute alcoholic hepatitis, 43, 83, 84, 85, 86, 89, 95
acute rejection, 83
adaptive immunity, 24
adenine, 8, 35, 65, 110
adenosine, ix, 32, 34, 35, 37, 39, 41, 44, 47, 48, 112, 132, 139
adenosine triphosphate, 112
adenovirus, 27
adhesion, 36
adipose tissue, 56
adolescents, 106
adults, 64, 66, 68, 95
Advanced Composition Tests, 57
adverse effects, 73
aerobic exercise, 107
aerodigestive tract, 90
age, 72, 85, 86
aggregation, 113
agonist, 39
alanine aminotransferase, viii, 2, 11, 72, 106
albumin, 54, 71
albuminuria, 102
alcohol abuse, vii, viii, x, 2, 9, 10, 11, 12, 32, 52, 65, 66, 67, 72, 76, 82, 102, 109
alcohol consumption, 4, 6, 7, 9, 11, 15, 21, 23, 24, 25, 29, 39, 64, 71, 73, 75, 80, 87, 88, 97, 104, 112
alcohol dehydrogenase (ADH), 3, 4, 5, 6, 11, 12, 13, 14, 15, 65, 103, 104, 110, 112, 120, 124, 125, 137, 143, 150, 152, 153, 154, 155, 156, 157, 158
alcohol dependence, 76, 88, 89, 112
alcohol use, 23, 42, 52, 66, 69, 71, 75, 80, 81, 87, 88, 97
alcohol withdrawal, 75, 86
alcoholic cirrhosis, x, 57, 58, 68, 69, 74, 79, 80, 81, 82, 83, 85, 86, 87, 88, 92, 94, 95, 96, 99, 116
alcoholic liver disease, vii, viii, ix, x, 1, 2, 4, 6, 7, 9, 10, 11, 12, 14, 15, 16, 17, 18, 19, 21, 23, 24, 25, 26, 27, 28, 31, 32, 34, 37, 42, 43, 44, 45, 46, 51, 52, 53, 58, 59, 60, 63, 64, 65, 66, 67, 68, 69, 70, 71, 72, 73, 74, 75, 76, 77, 79, 80, 81, 82, 83, 86, 88, 91, 92, 93, 94, 95, 96, 97, 98, 102, 103, 104, 106, 107, 109, 112, 116, 117, 119, 122, 140, 142, 146, 147, 148, 152, 153, 154, 157, 158

alcoholics, x, 4, 6, 11, 14, 21, 23, 63, 64, 66, 67, 68, 70, 71, 72, 73, 76, 80, 89
alcoholism, 5, 21, 25, 64, 73, 76, 80, 86, 89, 93, 116
aldehyde dehydrogenase, 3, 5, 14, 111, 137, 143
algorithm, 84
allele, 5, 6, 112
ALT, viii, 2, 11, 39, 72, 103
alters, 45
amino, x, 11, 63
amino acid(s), x, 63
amiodarone, 102
antagonism, 48
antibody, 21, 24
antigen, 12, 28
antigen-presenting cell, 28
anti-inflammatory agents, 105
antioxidant, 67, 69, 75
apoptosis, viii, 2, 10, 11, 14, 15, 16, 21, 22, 23, 27, 37, 46, 104, 130, 138, 141, 144, 145, 147, 148
appetite, 52
arrest, 22
artery, 115
aryl hydrocarbon receptor, 34
ascites, 25, 52, 54, 55, 56, 57, 58, 80
ascorbic acid, 68
aspartate, 11, 72, 106
assessment, vii, ix, 51, 52, 53, 56, 58, 59, 60, 61, 65, 82, 94
ATP, ix, 3, 6, 7, 8, 32, 33, 34, 35, 36, 37, 38, 39, 41, 42, 43, 44, 45, 47, 112, 120, 127, 129, 130, 131, 132, 133, 140, 141, 154, 156
atrophy, 55
autopsy, 106

B

bacteria, 19, 39, 104, 105, 114
barriers, 33
basement membrane, 114
Bcl-2 proteins, 10
behaviors, 89, 98
benefits, 24, 66
benign, 81, 102, 104
beta-carotene, 69
beverages, 104
BIA, 57, 58
bias, 88, 90, 93
bile duct, 114
bilirubin, 12, 92
binge drinking, 46, 87
biochemistry, 13
biomarkers, 16
biopsy, 16, 80, 103
bleeding, 52, 70, 80
blindness, 69, 72
blood, 13, 25, 65, 71, 75, 114
body composition, 57, 60, 76
body fat, 56
body mass index (BMI), 54, 102, 103
body weight, 11, 72
bone, 2, 37, 46, 70, 72
bone form, 72
bone marrow, 2, 37, 46
bowel, 26, 103, 110
brain, 25, 71
Brazil, 31
breakdown, 68

C

Ca^{2+}, 112
caffeine, 41
calcium, 71
calorie, x, 58, 59, 101
cancer, 6
candidates, 82, 85, 86, 88
CAP, 106
carbohydrate(s), vii, 1, 3, 6, 8, 13, 106
carbohydrate metabolism, 13
carbon, 3, 7, 28
carbon atoms, 7
carbon dioxide, 3, 7
carbon tetrachloride, 28
carboxylic acid, 6
cardiovascular disease, 88
carotene, 69, 76

cascades, 19
caspases, viii, 2, 145
catabolism, 5, 36, 37
caucasian population, 6
CD39, 34, 35, 36, 37, 44, 45
CD73, 35, 36, 37, 40, 44, 48
cell cycle, 22
cell death, 10, 11, 14, 15, 27
cell line(s), 26, 34, 49
cell surface, 35
CH3COOH, 5
challenges, 86
checks and balances, vii, viii, 1
chemokines, 36
chemotaxis, 36, 40, 44
children, 88
cholecalciferol, 70
cholestasis, 68, 115
cholesterol, 39
choline, 104
chronic active hepatitis, 21
chronic diseases, 36
circulation, 19, 22, 24, 33, 104, 112, 114
cirrhosis, ix, x, 21, 22, 23, 24, 25, 31, 32, 40, 41, 48, 49, 53, 54, 56, 59, 60, 61, 64, 71, 73, 80, 81, 82, 83, 84, 85, 86, 87, 90, 91, 92, 96, 101, 102, 103, 104, 105, 106, 109, 110, 113, 115
classes, 5
cleavage, 38
climate, 84
clinical judgment, 59
clinical presentation, x, 101
clinical trials, 33, 81, 93
clusters, 10
coagulopathy, 70
cobalamin, 67, 68
coding, 112
coenzyme, 66
coffee, 41, 49, 104
collagen, 40, 41, 49, 69, 114
coma, 14
competition, 69
complement, 21, 22
compliance, 82, 87, 88, 95
complications, 52, 56, 71, 72, 73, 90, 98
composition, 57, 58
compounds, 47
concordance, 36
condensation, 10
conduction, 57
conference, 82, 95
conflict of interest, 89
consensus, 52, 59, 82, 91, 93
constituents, 8, 112
consumption, vii, viii, x, 1, 2, 5, 14, 41, 46, 52, 53, 71, 80, 87, 89, 97, 101, 110, 113
consumption patterns, 97
control group, 84
controversial, vii, x, 2, 39, 79, 81, 84, 88, 90
coordination, 44
cornea, 5
correlation, 6, 54, 56
corticosteroids, 42, 81
cost, 42
counseling, 88, 90
CPT, 80, 81, 84, 86
creatine, 55
creatinine, 54, 57, 58, 60
crystals, 37, 39, 40, 45
currency, 34
current limit, 83
cytochrome, 4, 10, 13, 69, 103, 110, 112
cytokines, 19, 20, 21, 22, 23, 34, 36, 37, 38, 45, 46, 104
cytoplasm, 10, 111, 112
cytoskeleton, 112, 113
cytotoxicity, 73

D

damages, vii, 104
danger, ix, 20, 27, 32, 33, 34, 36, 37, 38, 39, 41, 42, 43, 44, 45
database, 85, 95, 107
deaths, 88, 91
deficiencies, 53, 64
deficiency, 5, 38, 60, 64, 65, 66, 67, 68, 69, 70, 71, 72, 73, 74, 75, 76, 103
degradation, 65

dendritic cell(s), viii, 17, 18, 36
deposition, 40, 105
derivatives, 34
destruction, 112
detection, 25, 47, 75
detoxification, 18
diabetes, 103, 104, 105, 107
diarrhea, 71
diet, 38, 39, 53, 67, 105, 106
dietary intake, x, 60, 63, 64, 65, 66, 67, 68, 70, 71
direct bilirubin, 12
disease(s), vii, viii, ix, x, 1, 2, 4, 6, 7, 9, 10, 11, 12, 14, 15, 16, 17, 18, 21, 22, 23, 24, 25, 26, 27, 28, 29, 31, 32, 33, 34, 37, 38, 42, 43, 44, 45, 46, 48, 51, 52, 53, 55, 56, 57, 58, 59, 61, 63, 64, 65, 66, 67, 68, 69, 70, 71, 72, 73, 74, 75, 76, 79, 80, 82, 83, 86, 87, 88, 91, 92, 93, 94, 95, 96, 97, 98, 99, 101, 102, 103, 104, 105, 106, 107, 109, 112, 116, 117, 120, 121, 122, 130, 140, 141, 142, 143, 144, 146, 147, 148, 149, 152, 153, 154, 155, 157, 158
disease progression, ix, 32, 33, 105
distribution, 5, 10, 57, 117
DNA, 8, 14, 16, 20, 25, 46, 67, 68, 111, 112
drug abuse, 98
drugs, 13, 102, 105
duodenum, 4, 71
DWI, 60
dyslipidemia, 102

E

edema, 54, 55, 56, 57
editors, 74, 116
electron(s), 4, 7, 8, 9, 14, 110, 113
electron microscopy, 14, 113
emergency, 76
employment, 83, 94
encephalopathy, 64, 72, 76
encoding, 112
endothelium, 36
endotoxemia, 26, 42, 73
endotoxins, 9, 114
energy, 3, 7, 8, 20, 34, 51, 52, 53, 56, 57, 58, 110
energy expenditure, 59
environment, 19, 20, 23, 37, 71, 110, 112
environmental factors, 83
enzyme(s), viii, 2, 3, 4, 5, 8, 11, 35, 65, 66, 68, 71, 110, 112
epidemiology, 91
epigenetics, 107
epithelium, 19
epitopes, 29
ergocalciferol, 70
esophageal varices, 24
esophagus, 6
ethanol, vii, viii, 1, 2, 4, 7, 9, 11, 13, 15, 19, 20, 21, 24, 25, 26, 27, 28, 29, 38, 40, 43, 46, 48, 74, 76, 97, 103, 110, 112, 113, 116, 117
ethanol metabolism, viii, 2, 116
ethanol-mediated liver injury, 29, 151
ethical implications, 86
ethnicity, 104
etiology, 80, 102
eukaryotic, 7
eukaryotic cell, 7
Europe, 82, 84, 94
evidence, vii, viii, 2, 11, 12, 49, 52, 53, 65, 68, 70, 76, 85, 86, 88, 101, 103
evolution, 14
excretion, 54, 57, 67, 68, 71, 72
exercise, 102, 105
exposure, 9, 19, 26, 33, 41, 43, 46, 67, 70, 104, 110, 111
extracellular matrix, 21, 22, 114
extracellular nucleotides, ix, 32, 36

F

FAD, 65
family history, 104, 107
family members, 85
fat, vii, x, 4, 6, 21, 52, 53, 55, 56, 57, 63, 64, 68, 69, 101, 102, 103, 104, 105, 107, 109, 111, 112, 123, 124, 156
fat soluble, x, 63, 64, 69

fatty acids, viii, 1, 3, 6, 13, 20, 102, 104
fetal alcohol syndrome, 6
fiber, 104
fibroblasts, 40, 114
fibrogenesis, 28, 48, 114
fibrosis, ix, x, 11, 16, 19, 20, 21, 22, 23, 26, 28, 31, 32, 38, 40, 41, 45, 48, 66, 69, 71, 73, 101, 103, 104, 105, 107, 109, 110, 114
filtration, 102
flora, 26
fluctuations, 54
fluid, 10, 52, 53, 54, 57, 112
folate, 66, 67, 74
folic acid, 67
food, vii, 3, 5, 8, 53, 102
food habits, 53
force, 8
formation, 6, 8, 34, 64, 65, 67, 71
formula, 81
fragments, 11
France, 84
free radicals, 27, 69, 71
fructose, 103
functional changes, 40

G

GABA, 66
gastric mucosa, 4
gastrointestinal tract, 19, 73, 110
gender differences, 4
gene expression, 28, 37
generalizability, 89
genes, 5, 33, 73, 112, 116
genetic factors, 102
genetics, 14, 104
genome, 104
glucose, vii, 1, 3, 4, 7, 8, 103
glutamate, 5, 67
glutamic acid, 66
glutamine, 25
glutathione, 13, 65, 66, 72, 111
glycerol, 6, 111
glycogen, 6, 102
glycolysis, 6, 7
gout, 37
guidelines, 76, 95

H

half-life, 44
Hand Grip Strength (HGS), 55, 61
healing, 41
health, 24, 27, 91, 93, 110
heavy drinking, 90
height, 54, 61
hemorrhage, 85
hepatic encephalopathy, 52, 72, 73, 80
hepatic fibrosis, 14, 26, 41, 48, 69
hepatic injury, 110, 112
hepatic necrosis, 43
hepatic neutrophil infiltration, 28, 29
hepatic stellate cells, 19, 21, 22, 28, 40, 41, 48
hepatitis, viii, ix, x, 2, 11, 12, 16, 20, 21, 23, 28, 29, 31, 32, 33, 42, 43, 45, 52, 59, 70, 73, 75, 79, 80, 81, 83, 84, 85, 86, 90, 92, 93, 94, 95, 102, 104, 105, 106, 107, 109, 110, 113, 115
hepatitis a, ix, x, 12, 31, 81, 84, 85, 95, 109
hepatitis c, 11, 93
hepatitis d, 70
hepatocellular cancer, ix, 31, 32
hepatocellular carcinoma (HCC), x, 21, 29, 40, 67, 101, 102, 103, 105, 106, 107, 110
hepatocytes, viii, x, 2, 4, 10, 11, 12, 13, 16, 19, 20, 21, 22, 23, 27, 38, 40, 43, 103, 104, 109, 110, 111, 112, 113, 114, 115
hepatorenal syndrome, 55
hepatotoxicity, viii, 2, 12, 27, 65
heterogeneity, 81
hispanics, 104
histology, x, 89, 101, 102, 104
histones, 8
history, 12, 52, 53, 86, 88, 89, 90, 91, 105
homeostasis, 6, 71
homocysteine, 66, 67, 75
hormones, 67
hospitalization, 69

host, viii, 17, 18, 22, 34, 38, 47, 48
human, ix, 14, 15, 18, 19, 23, 25, 26, 33, 38, 44, 71, 72, 104, 116, 117
human neutrophils, 44
human subjects, 19, 72
hyaline, 84, 112
hydrogen, 5, 8
hydrogen peroxide, 5
hyperinsulinemia, 103
hyperlipidemia, 104
hypertension, 92, 102
hypoglycemia, 6
hypomagnesemia, 71
hypoparathyroidism, 71
hypothesis, 104
hypoxia, 34, 44, 104

I

IFNγ, 22, 23
IL-1, ix, 22, 32, 36, 37, 38, 39, 41, 46, 104
IL-17, 22
IL-1β, ix, 32, 36, 37, 38, 39, 41
IL-6, 22, 28, 33, 34, 37, 149
IL-8, 22, 33, 37, 44
immune function, 72
immune reaction, 10
immune system, 15, 19, 24, 33, 34, 46, 104
immunity, 33, 42
immunohistochemistry, 12
immunomodulatory, 37
immunosuppression, 82, 90
immunosuppressive therapies, viii, 2
impaired immune function, 69, 70
in vitro, 40, 107
in vivo, 45, 58
incidence, 65, 76, 83, 98, 105
individuals, ix, 46, 51, 53, 54, 55, 64, 103, 110
inducer, ix, 18
inducible enzyme, 4
induction, 20, 33, 40, 44, 46
infection, viii, 12, 17, 18, 21, 33, 47, 94, 107
inflammasome, ix, 20, 27, 31, 32, 33, 34, 36, 37, 38, 39, 40, 41, 42, 44, 45, 46, 47, 48, 107
inflammation, viii, ix, 15, 17, 18, 19, 20, 22, 23, 24, 25, 31, 32, 33, 34, 36, 37, 38, 39, 40, 41, 43, 44, 45, 47, 104, 105, 110, 114
inflammatory cells, 10, 19, 23, 114
inflammatory responses, 21, 24, 45
infliximab, 43
ingestion, x, 5, 71, 80, 83, 101
inhibition, 7, 36, 40
inhibitor, 34, 41, 44
initiation, 9, 10, 81
injury, viii, x, 2, 9, 12, 15, 17, 18, 19, 20, 21, 22, 23, 26, 27, 28, 29, 32, 36, 37, 39, 40, 42, 43, 45, 46, 48, 64, 68, 69, 71, 72, 74, 75, 76, 77, 80, 81, 104, 109, 110, 112, 114, 117
innate immune response(s), 36, 44
innate immunity, 27, 36, 45
insulation, 9
insulin, 27, 71, 102, 103, 105
insulin resistance, 27, 71, 102, 104
integrity, vii, viii, 2, 9, 13
interface, 114
interferon, 22
intervention, 58, 90
intestine, 64, 67, 116
iron, 70, 71, 76, 125, 128, 145, 148
ischemia, 15
Israel, 1, 29, 51, 63, 79, 101, 109
issues, 76, 82, 89, 110

J

jaundice, 80, 81, 85
jejunum, 110

K

ketoacidosis, 14
kidney, 70, 89, 98
kidney transplantation, 89
kill, 22

Krebs cycle, 110
Kupffer cells, viii, 17, 18, 19, 20, 21, 22, 23, 24, 27, 33, 41, 43, 46, 114, 117, 144

L

labeling, 12
lactic acid, 6
Lactobacillus, 26
latency, viii, 2, 9, 10, 11
leakage, viii, 2, 8
leaks, 67
lean body mass, 55, 56, 57
lesions, 110
lifetime, 89
ligand, 22, 35, 38
light, 14, 32, 84, 104
lipid peroxidation, 69, 111
lipids, x, 3, 8, 24, 25, 63, 112
liver, vii, viii, ix, x, 1, 2, 3, 4, 5, 6, 7, 8, 9, 10, 11, 13, 14, 15, 17, 18, 19, 20, 21, 22, 23, 24, 25, 26, 27, 28, 29, 31, 32, 33, 36, 37, 38, 39, 40, 41, 42, 43, 44, 46, 48, 49, 51, 52, 53, 54, 55, 56, 57, 58, 59, 60, 61, 64, 65, 66, 67, 68, 69, 70, 71, 72, 73, 74, 75, 76, 77, 79, 80, 81, 82, 84, 85, 86, 89, 91, 92, 93, 94, 95, 96, 97, 98, 99, 101, 102, 103, 104, 105, 106, 107, 109, 110, 112, 114, 117
liver cancer, 41, 107
liver cells, viii, 2, 9, 11, 13, 46
liver cirrhosis, 23, 59, 60, 80
liver damage, viii, 2, 7, 38, 39, 104, 112
liver disease, vii, ix, 1, 2, 6, 9, 10, 11, 21, 23, 24, 27, 28, 29, 31, 32, 38, 42, 44, 48, 51, 52, 53, 55, 56, 57, 58, 59, 61, 66, 67, 68, 69, 70, 71, 72, 73, 74, 75, 86, 91, 92, 102, 103, 104, 105, 106, 107, 112
liver enzymes, 26
liver failure, 40, 84
liver inflammation, ix, 31, 33
liver transplant, vii, x, 40, 59, 79, 82, 93, 94, 95, 96, 97, 98, 99, 105
liver transplantation, vii, x, 40, 59, 79, 82, 83, 87, 91, 93, 94, 95, 96, 97, 98, 99
localization, 116
lung cancer, 76
lymphocytes, viii, 17, 18, 21, 22
lysine, 5
lysis, 112

M

macronutrients, 53
macrophage inflammatory protein, 45
macrophages, viii, 11, 17, 18, 20, 21, 22, 28, 33, 36, 37, 39, 44, 45
magnesium, 71
magnitude, 19
majority, 51, 82, 88, 103, 104
malabsorption, x, 52, 63, 64, 70
malaria, 22
malignancy, x, 79, 87, 90, 98
malignant tumors, 88
malnutrition, ix, x, 33, 51, 52, 53, 54, 55, 56, 58, 59, 60, 61, 63, 64, 71, 76, 121, 143
management, x, 42, 73, 75, 79, 81, 84, 86, 89, 91, 95, 96, 106
Maryland, 91
mass, 55, 56, 57, 59, 60, 105
matrix, 7, 8, 40, 114
measurement(s), 55, 56, 57, 76, 116
median, 84
Medicaid, 82
medical, x, 52, 79, 81, 82, 83, 85, 86, 88
medical care, 82
Medicare, 82, 107
medicine, 26, 28, 93, 95, 96, 116
membrane permeability, 33, 41
membranes, 7, 9, 10, 112, 114
mental capacity, 53
metabolic, 14, 43, 47, 74, 102, 105, 107
metabolic acidosis, 6
metabolic syndrome, 103, 104, 105
metabolism, vii, 1, 2, 3, 4, 6, 7, 8, 9, 10, 11, 12, 13, 18, 33, 44, 52, 66, 69, 70, 72, 73, 74, 76, 104, 110, 112, 116
metabolites, viii, ix, 1, 20, 23, 26, 32, 33, 34, 69, 103, 110

metabolized, vii, 2, 103, 110, 111
metabolizing, 4
metabolome, 24
metformin, 105
methodology, 91
methylation, 65, 67
mice, 15, 22, 26, 27, 28, 38, 39, 40, 42, 46, 48, 77
microbiota, 15, 105
microorganisms, 19
microRNA, 44
microsomal ethanol-oxidizing system, 4
microsomes, 110
Mid-arm Circumference (MAC), 56
migration, 36, 41, 45, 48
misuse, 73, 75
mitochondria, vii, viii, 1, 2, 3, 5, 6, 7, 8, 9, 10, 11, 12, 13, 14, 34, 103, 110, 111, 115, 119, 120, 122, 126, 127, 128, 129, 130, 131, 133, 134, 136, 137, 139, 141, 142, 145, 146, 147, 148, 150, 152, 155, 156
mitochondrial damage, vii, viii, 2, 4, 7, 103, 111
mitochondrial DNA, viii, 2, 8, 37
models, ix, 9, 32, 34, 71, 80
modern society, 104
molecular weight, 5
molecules, 6, 7, 18, 19, 34, 36, 37, 39, 111
monoclonal antibody, 43
morbidity, 89, 90
mortality, ix, x, 31, 32, 45, 56, 60, 68, 69, 70, 73, 79, 80, 81, 86, 89, 90, 91, 92, 94, 109
mortality rate, 80
motivation, 82
mRNA, 44, 48, 73
mtDNA, vii, viii, 2, 8, 9, 10, 12
mucosa, 25
multiple factors, 110
multivariate analysis, 81
muscle, 2, 7, 52, 53, 54, 55, 56, 58, 60, 61, 71
muscle mass, 53, 54, 55, 60, 61
muscle strength, 54
mutant, 5
mutation(s), 5, 14
myeloid cells, 36
myofibroblasts, 28, 115

N

NAD, vii, 3, 4, 5, 6, 7, 65, 110, 111
NADH, 3, 4, 6, 7, 8, 9, 65, 110, 111
National Academy of Sciences, 27
National Institutes of Health, 91, 93
natural killer (NK) cells, viii, 17, 18
natural killer T cells, 28, 29
necrosis, 10, 20, 21, 27, 43, 112, 114
neurotransmitter, 66
neutrophils, 20, 23, 28, 36, 44, 113
New England, 93, 95, 106
NFk-B, 33
niacin, 65, 74
nicotinamide, 65, 110
nicotinic acid, 75
nitrogen, 54
NK cells, 23
NLRP3, 36, 37, 38, 39, 40, 44
nonalcoholic steatohepatitis (NASH), 9, 26, 101, 102, 103, 104, 105, 106, 107, 148, 157
nuclear receptors, 74
nuclei, 111, 112
nucleotides, ix, 32, 36
nucleus, 10, 103, 111, 112
nutrient(s), x, 3, 18, 52, 53, 63, 75, 105
nutrition, vii, ix, 51, 52, 53, 55, 56, 58, 59, 61, 75, 102
nutritional assessment, 58, 59
nutritional deficiencies, 55, 76
nutritional state, 57, 59
nutritional status, 56, 59

O

obesity, 102, 103, 104, 106
organ(s), viii, x, 2, 3, 17, 18, 84, 86, 87, 109, 110

organelle(s), 7, 10, 11, 112
organism, 10
osteoporosis, 70, 71
outpatient(s), 52, 53, 55, 59
overweight, 105
oxidation, vii, 2, 3, 4, 6, 7, 8, 9, 59, 65, 69, 102, 110, 111
oxidative damage, 8
oxidative phosphorylation, 8, 112, 129, 132, 133, 141
oxidative reaction, 34
oxidative stress, 20, 28, 33, 34, 68, 69, 71, 72, 73, 75, 77, 103
oxygen, viii, 2, 4, 8, 9, 21, 112

P

pancreas, 2, 7
pancreatic insufficiency, 68, 69, 70
paracentesis, 54
parallel, 71, 113
parathyroid hormone, 71
pathogenesis, ix, 15, 18, 21, 22, 27, 28, 32, 39, 40, 41, 42, 48
pathogens, viii, 17, 18, 20, 36, 39
pathology, 14, 19, 25
pathophysiology, viii, ix, 2, 4, 19, 24, 32, 105
pathway(s), vii, 3, 4, 5, 6, 21, 24, 25, 26, 47, 72, 110
pattern recognition, 37
pellagra, 65
pentoxifylline, viii, 2, 12, 16, 93, 107, 144
peripheral neuropathy, 66
permeability, 9, 15, 23, 25, 28, 42, 104, 107, 112, 113
phagocytic cells, 22
phagocytosis, 15
pharmacokinetics, 13
pharmacology, 91, 93
phosphate, 66, 102
phosphorylation, 8, 112
physical activity, 53, 55, 104
physical assessment, 52, 55, 61
physicians, 76, 86
physiology, 19, 25, 26
pigs, 67, 73
pilot study, 26
placebo, 70, 71, 75
plasma levels, 19
poison, 102
polymorphism(s), 104, 112
population, viii, 17, 18, 51, 55, 56, 70, 85, 102, 103, 105, 106
portal hypertension, 40, 91
portal vein, 103, 115
positive correlation, 56
post-transplant, x, 79, 83, 84, 85, 86, 87, 88, 89, 90
prednisone, 81
prevention, 73, 75, 89
probiotics, 19, 104, 105
prognosis, 80, 81, 88, 92, 93
pro-inflammatory, 20, 29, 36, 37
proliferation, 5
promoter, 112
protection, 25, 39
protective role, 22, 23, 41
protein synthesis, 52, 54
proteins, 3, 5, 8, 9, 10, 21, 24, 39, 44, 46, 54, 67, 75, 112, 113, 114
protons, 8
pseudomonas aeruginosa, 39, 47
psychiatric disorder(s), 85
psychologist, 88
psychosocial factors, 88
psychosomatic, 88
public support, 84
purinergic signaling, ix, 31, 32, 34, 35, 44
pyridoxine, 66

Q

quality of life, 83, 95

R

race, 86
radicals, 21, 69

reactions, vii, 3, 6, 65, 67
reactive oxygen, vii, 4, 8, 12, 20
recall, 53, 88
receptor(s), ix, 19, 21, 26, 32, 33, 34, 35, 36, 37, 38, 39, 40, 46, 47, 48, 113
recidivism, x, 79, 82, 84, 85, 87, 88, 89, 90, 96
recidivism rate, 89
recognition, 23, 29, 47, 48
recommendations, 58, 91
recovery, 12, 86
recurrence, 99
recycling, 55
redundancy, viii, 2, 8, 10, 11
regeneration, ix, 17, 18, 33, 40, 68
regenerative capacity, viii, 2
registry, 83, 94
regression, 48
rehabilitation, 82, 88
rehabilitation program, 82
rejection, 83
relevance, 5, 104
reliability, 56
renal dysfunction, 55
renal failure, 81, 93
repair, ix, 8, 17, 18, 28, 37
repressor, 33
requirement(s), 7, 9, 82
reserves, 56
resistance, 22, 57, 102
resolution, 22, 37
response, ix, 17, 18, 19, 22, 27, 32, 36, 37, 39, 40, 44, 47, 68, 104
restoration, 24
reticulum, 4, 110
retinol, 68
riboflavin, 65, 76
risk, x, 5, 12, 42, 51, 54, 58, 60, 67, 68, 69, 70, 79, 80, 81, 82, 83, 85, 87, 88, 89, 90, 91, 96, 98, 101, 102, 103, 104, 105, 106, 107
risk factors, x, 51, 90, 96, 101, 102, 104, 106
RNA, 20, 47
rodents, 21, 25

S

Salmonella, 39
saturated fat(s), 20, 104, 105
saturated fatty acids, 20
saturation, 71
secrete, 114
secretion, 36, 47, 68, 107
sensing, 38
sensitivity, 26, 34, 53, 55, 105, 112
sensitization, 26, 34
sepsis, 34
serum, viii, 2, 11, 12, 33, 37, 38, 43, 46, 54, 65, 67, 68, 69, 70, 71, 106
serum albumin, 54
sex, 85
shock, 44, 113
shortage, 84
showing, 41
side effects, 42
signals, ix, 20, 27, 32, 33, 34, 35, 38, 39, 41, 42, 43, 44, 102
signs, 51, 55, 58
skeletal muscle, 60, 71
skin, 56
small intestine, x, 4, 63, 64, 66, 67
smoking, 89, 90, 98
sobriety, 88
social support, 82, 88
socioeconomic background, 85
specialists, 87, 89
species, vii, viii, 2, 4, 8, 12, 20
spectroscopy, 106
starvation, 55, 60
state(s), 6, 80, 89
stellate cells, 19, 21, 22, 27, 28, 40, 41, 48, 49, 69, 73, 114
stenosis, 90
sterile, 18, 27, 33, 39, 42, 44
steroids, viii, 2, 12, 92, 105, 126
stimulation, 23, 34, 44, 45, 72
stomach, 4, 5, 103, 110, 116
storage, 3, 105
stress, viii, 1, 34
stressors, 34

structural changes, viii, 2, 10
structural gene, 8
structure, 7, 8, 9, 12
substance abuse, 89, 117
substance use, 88
substitution, 5
substrate(s), vii, 8, 13, 20, 59
Sun, 14, 45, 75
supplementation, 58, 65, 66, 67, 68, 69, 70, 71, 72, 73, 74, 75, 77
suppression, 36
surplus, 9
surveillance, x, 79, 90, 99
survival, 12, 80, 81, 82, 83, 84, 85, 86, 87, 90, 91, 92, 94, 96, 97, 99
survival rate, 80, 81, 83, 85, 87
sweat, 4
swelling, 10, 11
symptoms, 38, 53, 65, 81
syndrome, 64, 75, 76, 102, 103, 105, 107
synthesis, 4, 6, 8, 21, 37, 38, 67, 68, 102, 110

T

T cell(s), 23, 24, 28, 29
Taiwan, 107
Tamoxifen, 102
target, viii, 17, 18, 48, 87
Task Force, 59
techniques, 57
testing, 55
TGF, 26, 40, 41
therapeutic effect(s), 24
therapeutic targets, 42
therapeutics, 91, 93
therapy, 32, 43, 45, 52, 70, 74, 76, 81, 83, 84, 92
Thiamine, 64, 73, 74, 75, 76, 144
thrombosis, 90
time periods, 87
tissue, viii, 5, 9, 10, 11, 17, 18, 25, 37, 39, 40, 57, 68, 69, 71, 73, 84, 111
TLR4, 19, 20, 21, 26, 27, 33, 37, 38
TNF-alpha, 26, 28, 44
TNF-α, 33, 37, 38, 113
tobacco, x, 79, 87, 89, 90
Toll-like receptor (TLR), 19, 23, 26, 36, 39, 45, 46
toxic effect, 9, 69
toxic products, 33
toxicity, ix, 2, 18, 66
toxin, 10, 110
trafficking, 44
training, 107
transaminases, viii, 2, 103
transcription, 21, 76
transcription factors, 76
transferrin, 71, 103, 106
translation, 33
translocation, 15, 19, 23, 25, 33, 46, 104
transplant, x, 79, 81, 82, 83, 84, 86, 87, 88, 89, 90, 94
transplant recipients, 84
transplantation, 32, 83, 84, 86, 88, 90, 91, 93, 94, 95, 96, 97, 98, 99
transport, 4, 7, 8, 9, 71
trauma, 34
treatment, viii, ix, x, 2, 20, 31, 32, 34, 36, 39, 72, 73, 75, 76, 79, 81, 84, 86, 89, 97, 107
trial, 43, 71, 75, 76, 81, 93, 96
tricarboxylic acid cycle, 20
tricep skinfold test, 56
triggers, viii, 2, 10, 19, 21, 33
triglycerides, 6, 102, 105, 111
tryptophan, 65
tumo(u)r(s), viii, 2, 5, 24, 28, 43, 44, 45, 90
tumor necrosis factor (TNF), viii, 2, 26, 28, 33, 37, 38,43, 44, 45, 104, 113
tumours, 24
type 2 diabetes, 106

U

ubiquitin, 113
unconjugated bilirubin, 34
undernutrition, 60
United States (USA), 27, 32, 58, 64, 66, 74, 80, 82, 83, 84, 91, 93, 102, 107

uric acid, ix, 32, 33, 37, 38, 39, 41, 42, 43, 45
urinary tract, 98
urine, 4, 65

V

vacuole, 111
vasculature, 34
venules, 110
virus infection, 21, 28
viruses, 19, 20
visceral adiposity, 107
vitamin A, 68, 69, 72, 73
vitamin B1, 68, 73
vitamin B12, 68, 73
Vitamin C, 68, 74
vitamin D, 70, 71
vitamin D deficiency, 70, 71
vitamin E, 69, 70, 74, 75, 76, 105, 136, 145
vitamin supplementation, vii
vitamins, x, 63, 64, 68, 69, 75, 128, 143
VLDL, 102, 107, 112

W

Washington, 74
waste, 7
wasting, 52, 55, 56
water, 3, 4, 54, 57, 61
weakness, 55, 60
weight changes, 57
weight loss, 53
withdrawal, 66, 98

Y

yeast, 105
yield, 3

Z

zinc, 5, 72, 73
zinc sulfate, 72